Discussions in Patient Management

TUBERCULOSIS

By

DOUGLAS R. GRACEY, M.S., M.D., F.A.C.P., F.C.C.P.
Consultant in Thoracic Diseases and Intensive Respiratory Care
Mayo Clinic;
Associate Professor of Medicine
Mayo Medical School
Rochester, Minnesota

and

WHITNEY W. ADDINGTON, M.S., M.D., F.A.C.P., F.C.C.P.
Chairman, Division of Pulmonary Medicine
Cook County Hospital;
Associate Professor of Medicine
University of Illinois Medical School
Chicago, Illinois

Medical Examination Publishing Co., Inc.
an Excerpta Medica company

969 Stewart Avenue • Garden City, New York 11530

Library of Congress Card Number
79-88043

ISBN 0-87488-875-1

May, 1979

Printed in the United States of America

SIMULTANEOUSLY PUBLISHED IN:

Europe	:	HANS HUBER PUBLISHERS Bern, Switzerland
Mexico, Central America, and South America (except Brazil)	:	EDITORIAL EL MANUAL MODERNO Mexico City, Mexico
South and East Asia	:	TOPPAN COMPANY (S) Pte. Ltd. Singapore
United Kingdom	:	HENRY KIMPTON PUBLISHERS London, England

PREFACE

This book is written for the physician who is not trained in pulmonary medicine, infectious disease, or tuberculosis care. Tuberculosis, once a common medical problem, is now so rarely seen by most primary care physicians that they know little about the disease. In fact, many physicians do not think of tuberculosis when treating patients with classic chest roentgenographic changes. To compound the problem, tuberculosis must now be treated by the primary care physician, as most tuberculosis sanatoria have been closed. In order to accept this responsibility, the primary care physician must learn to diagnose tuberculosis and provide appropriate drug therapy. Our intention is to introduce the basic concepts of this diagnosis and treatment. Appropriate references are provided for the reader who wishes to pursue further in-depth study.

We wish to emphasize that the practice of tuberculosis chemotherapy is rapidly changing; and although we have stressed conventional concepts of treatment, we have also discussed newer methods. Many of the new methods of treatment appear to be as efficacious as the older standard forms of therapy; however, the physician who is not an expert in tuberculosis treatment is probably wise to follow the older, more conventional treatment regimens at the present time.

The Authors

DEDICATION

We dedicate this book to our wives, Edith and Ada; and to Areta Gracey, in memory of Warren R. Gracey, who fought the scourge of tuberculosis before chemotherapy changed the momentum of the battle.

ACKNOWLEDGMENTS

We acknowledge, with appreciation, the assistance of our secretaries, Mrs. Pennylu Marshall, Mrs. Ernestine Daniels, and Miss Ellen Graupmann.

Contents

I INTRODUCTION 1

II THE DIAGNOSIS OF TUBERCULOSIS 5
Tuberculin Skin Test 6
Cultures for Mycobacteria 7
Sputum 7
Gastric Washings 8
Pleural Fluid. 8
Urine 8
Tissue Aspirates and Body Fluids. 9

III TUBERCULIN SKIN TESTING AND PREVENTIVE THERAPY 13
Tuberculin Skin Testing. 13
Candidates for Preventive Therapy. 14
Contact Evaluation 18
BCG Vaccination 21

IV THE TREATMENT OF TUBERCULOSIS. 24
Principles of Chemotherapy 24
Drug Actions and Side Effects 25
The Practice of Chemotherapy 29
Categorization and Treatment 29
Discharge of Patients from Medical Surveillance . . 31
Treatment of Children 31
Complications of Tuberculosis 33
Extrapulmonary Tuberculosis 35
Miliary Tuberculosis 37
Corticosteroids as an Adjunct to Treatment 38
Supervised Intermittent Therapy 39
Illustrative Cases. 40

V RESISTANT TUBERCULOSIS 60
Retreatment for Resistant Disease. 64

VI THE MYCOBACTERIOSES 69
Skin Tests for Atypical Organisms 73
Illustrative Cases 77

VII SURGICAL THERAPY OF PULMONARY TUBERCULOSIS 87

APPENDICES

APPENDIX 1: Table I - Classification of Tuberculosis. . . 93

APPENDIX 2: Table II - Doses and Characteristics of Antituberculous Drugs 96

APPENDIX 3: Significant Drug Resistance Levels in Direct Drug Susceptibility Studies on 7H11 Media. . . 106

INDEX 111

notice

The editor(s) and/or author(s) and the publisher of this book have made every effort to ensure that all therapeutic modalities that are recommended are in accordance with accepted standards at the time of publication.

The drugs specified within this book may not have specific approval by the Food and Drug Administration in regard to the indications and dosages that are recommended by the editor(s) and/or author(s). The manufacturer's package insert is the best source of current prescribing information.

CHAPTER I:

INTRODUCTION

One of the most remarkable stories of modern medicine has been that of the conquest of tuberculosis. Marten, in 1720, wrote, "Of all the distempers that afflict mankind, there is not one for the cure of which more remedies have been appropriated and invented than for phthisis or consumption of the lungs."[1] Although most physicians in the United States conceive of the therapy of tuberculosis as rather "cut and dried", investigation continues in the areas of prevention, transmissability and treatment. At the outset, we must state that our concepts of this disease will certainly continue to change as time passes, and much of what we set down in these pages may soon become outmoded. Many types of treatment including diet, heliotherapy, bedrest, fresh air, surgery, pneumothorax and institutional care have been advocated; but at the present time, it is generally accepted that outpatient chemotherapy is the major tool in the treatment of tuberculosis. Our concept of adequate chemotherapy has continued to evolve as newer drugs have become available and experience with various drug combinations and schedules of administration have been investigated in a systematic manner.

Newer programs involving supervised intermittent multiple drug therapy, short-term therapy (less than the conventional eighteen to twenty-four months), limited hospitalization and complete outpatient therapy are presently being investigated. These "radical" changes in our approach have been warmly endorsed by some pulmonary physicians and castigated by others.[2, 3] Studies have suggested that adequate drug therapy of ambulatory, home-dwelling tuberculous patients is effective and does not appreciably increase the risk of infection of close family contacts.[4] Supervised intermittent drug therapy and short-course chemotherapy appear, from presently available reports, to be effective but are still generally not accepted by many physicians treating tuberculosis in the United States.[5, 6] It would appear that such programs are sufficiently effective, however, for application to the group of inner-city vagrant patients, others who prove to be difficult treatment problems and the vast reservoir of chronic infective patients the world over. We feel that any regimen which is of proven effectiveness and safety should be considered in the treatment of the individual patient, if that program appears to be the best alternative in our attempt to arrest active disease and prevent reactivation at a later time.

At present, we employ a daily regimen of two or three drugs for responsible patients. Conversely, supervised intermittent or short-term therapy may be much more appropriate in the patient who is not dependable or motivated to follow standard daily programs. It is very possible that twice-weekly, after a course of initial daily therapy, and short-course therapy will eventually be standard treatment for all patients with tuberculosis.

The schema for the classification of tuberculosis has recently been revised and terms such as minimal, moderately-advanced, far-advanced, active, inactive and quiescent no longer apply. Although much of the former terminology was useful in the prechemotherapy era, it appears to be less useful today. The new classification schedule for tuberculosis describes the location of the infection (organ), bacteriologic status, chemotherapeutic status and roentgenographic appearance.[7]

Adequate bacteriologic studies remain the key to the diagnosis and evaluation of the effects of chemotherapy in tuberculosis. The finest physician, with excellent roentgenologic facilities, is in serious trouble if he attempts to diagnose and treat tuberculosis without the support of a well-trained and dependable bacteriologist, capable of using the newest methods for staining and culturing mycobacteria. In the final analysis, the bacteriologic status of the patient remains the cornerstone of the diagnosis of tuberculosis and the evaluation of the effect of therapy. The advisability of performing drug sensitivity studies routinely on the mycobacterial isolates of all patients with tuberculosis is another area of great controversy. Recent experience has suggested that routine drug sensitivity testing in previously untreated tuberculous patients is of little value.[8] However, many excellent centers maintain that routine drug sensitivity screening is valuable. Although the pros and cons of routine drug testing in the bacteriologic laboratory continue to be argued, there is no doubt that the physician must have this capability available, if not routinely, at least for the patient in whom treatment has been a failure, retreatment is necessary, or reactivation has occurred.

Pulmonary and extrapulmonary tuberculosis, nontuberculous mycobacterial disease, treatment failure, reactivation of disease in previously treated patients and the difficult patient all present diverse and special problems for the physician. These problems frequently require the expertise of specially trained physicians, nurses, social workers and other medical personnel equipped to handle the particular challenge presented by the patient. Although most physicians treating tuberculosis may not have a staff of such magnitude readily available, such services and consultation can usually be obtained for the patient, if one seeks help.

The events of the past few years have moved the treatment of tuberculosis out of the sanatorium and into the office and general hospital. We feel that this has been an excellent improvement in tuberculosis therapy since the asymptomatic or mildly ill tuberculous patient does not require prolonged hospital care. The truly sick patient belongs in a general hospital and not in a sanatorium, which has a very restricted area of medical interest and capability.

This movement of the care of the tuberculous patient into the general hospital has created a whole new set of problems, however, which the medical community must try to solve.[9, 10] The long-standing misconceptions of nurses, physicians and administrators regarding infectiousness, isolation precautions, social implications, etc., must be corrected before tuberculosis can be adequately managed in most general hospitals. Last but not least, the general physician and internist must accept responsibility for the treatment of tuberculosis if this disease is to be adequately managed in the future. It will no longer be possible to exile the tuberculous patient to a special hospital, and treatment will ultimately be supervised at home and in the general hospital. It is imperative that general physicians and internists become well acquainted with the methods of diagnosing and treating tuberculosis and the complications of the disease and of the drug therapy, as this age-old problem returns from the sanatorium to the world of general medicine.

It is our hope that this monograph will be of aid to the physician who has not been trained in pulmonary medicine in his approach to the diagnosis, treatment, and care of the patient with tuberculosis. We will frequently use the case history format in our discussions, as we feel that this method best illustrates many of the facets of tuberculosis in the most concise manner. We will discuss the various aspects of tuberculosis from the point of view of currently accepted practices, while attempting to bring to the reader some of the newer concepts of treatment and areas of current controversy.

REFERENCES

1. Marten B: A New Theory of Consumption, More Especially of a Phthisis or Consumption of the Lungs. London, 1720, page 273.

2. Bates JG: Ambulatory treatment of tuberculosis--An idea whose time is come. Am Rev Respir Dis 109:317, 1974.

3. Oatway WH: Early discharge of patients with active tuberculosis. Am Rev Respir Dis 109:320, 1974.

4. Fox W: The chemotherapy and epidemiology of tuberculosis, some findings of general applicability from the tuberculosis chemotherapy center; Madras. Lancet 2:413, 1962.

5. American Thoracic Society: Intermittent therapy for adults with tuberculosis. Am Rev Respir Dis 110:374, 1974

6. Fox W, Mitchison DA: Short course chemotherapy for pulmonary tuberculosis. Am Rev Respir Dis 111:845, 1975.

7. Diagnostic Standards and Classification of Tuberculosis and other Mycobacterial Diseases. New York, American Lung Association, 1974, page 34.

8. Hong Kong Tuberculosis Treatment Services/British Medical Research Council Investigation: A study in Hong Kong to evaluate the role of pretreatment susceptibility tests in the selection of regimens of chemotherapy for tuberculosis. Am Rev Respir Dis 106:1, 1972.

9. MacGregor RR: A year's experience with tuberculosis in a private urban teaching hospital in the postsanatorium era. Am J Med 58:221, 1975.

10. Reichman LB: Tuberculosis Care: When and where? Annals of Int Med 80:402, 1974.

CHAPTER II:

THE DIAGNOSIS OF TUBERCULOSIS

INTRODUCTION

Tuberculosis may involve multiple organs of the body and lead to a variety of signs and symptoms. Other diseases may mimic tuberculosis and vice versa and, at times, the diagnosis may prove most difficult and frustrating. The first step in the diagnosis of tuberculosis is suspicion. Unfortunately, the degree of suspicion that tuberculosis may be responsible for, the patient's symptoms and chest roentgenographic abnormalities has decreased with the incidence of the disease.

The definitive diagnosis of a tuberculous infection requires the culture of viable organisms from secretions, tissue fluid or tissue. In certain cases, tissue biopsy specimens revealing typical, caseating granulomas containing acid-fast bacilli are sufficient for diagnosis, with or without positive mycobacterial cultures. Every effort must be made to establish a diagnosis on the basis of mycobacterial cultures; this requires a competent bacteriology laboratory capable of isolating and classifying these organisms.

Infection with Mycobacterium tuberculosis is acquired by inhalation of droplet nuclei containing the organisms distally into the bronchial tree at the level of the respiratory bronchiole or alveolus. It is thought that droplet nuclei smaller than 10 microns in diameter are capable of deposition in these distal airways because their small size allows them to remain airborne and pass into the small airways without being deposited on the mucous blanket of the tracheobronchial tree. Deposition on the mucous blanket will normally allow their removal by normal mucociliary action to the oropharynx, where they may be expectorated or swallowed.

When M. tuberculosis is deposited in the respiratory bronchiole or alveolus, it invades the pulmonary parenchyma and multiplies. In the susceptible host, immune mechanisms do not immediately become operative and organisms multiply for a period of time despite engulfment by phagocytic cells. The organisms may spread to local and regional lymphatics and throughout the body via the bloodstream. This initial spread of the organisms to other organs may subsequently lead to extrapulmonary disease. Apparently, the majority of individuals with primary tuberculous infection are able to recruit the necessary immunologic defenses to wall off the infection and hold it in abatement henceforth. Certain patients, especially children, develop a progressive primary infection. It is generally felt, however, that most progressive pulmonary tuberculosis is a result of reactivation of a prior infection. This reactivation is more common in the first year or so after the initial infection has occurred. The rationale behind preventive therapy with isoniazid is the reduction of the number of viable residual mycobacteria and concomitantly the likelihood of reactivation.

Delayed hypersensitivity, as manifested by the positive tuberculin skin test, may not appear for two to ten weeks after infection. It would appear, however, that acquired immunity to tuberculosis and delayed tuberculin hypersensitivity are separate immune responses directed toward different components of the mycobacterial cell wall.[1]

TUBERCULIN SKIN TEST

Although widely used as a diagnostic tool, the tuberculin skin test is frequently misused and misinterpreted. A positive tuberculin test does not confirm the presence of progressive or active tuberculosis, and a negative test does not exclude infection with M. tuberculosis. A major problem with the diagnostic use of the tuberculin skin test is misinterpretation of a negative test. The problem of absorption of antigen onto glass containers and glass and plastic syringes has been alleviated by the use of Tween 80 stabilized purified protein derivative (PPD) preparations and improved technique. It seems clear that some of the problems of "false-negative" tuberculin tests resulted, and may still occur, because of inactive antigen preparations and poor technique.

The incidence of "false-negative" tuberculin skin tests in infected patients has been variously reported to range from 1 to 15 percent. The higher rate of "false-negative" tests is reported in general hospital populations, which include many patients with one or more of the problems leading to skin test anergy for tuberculin. The factors that may lead to a negative tuberculin test in the presence of progressive tuberculosis include: overwhelming tuberculous infection (i. e. miliary disease); intercurrent disease such as leukemia, lymphoma, sarcoidosis or recent measles; acute bacterial infections with leukocytosis; therapy with immunosuppressive drugs such as steroids; advanced age; recent onset of disease, with inadequate time to develop delayed hypersensitivity; recent immunizations; pregnancy; and poor technique in skin testing. A negative tuberculin skin test must never be taken as absolute evidence that the patient does not have tuberculosis, even if the above listed situations do not exist.

The problem of the "false-positive" skin test also may confuse the evaluation of findings in the individual patient. Recent blood transfusion, repeated skin testing in the same area, and prior BCG vaccination may all produce a positive tuberculin skin test in the uninfected person. Skin tests may also be incorrectly interpreted as being positive by the inexperienced observer. Older patients with initial negative PPD skin tests may appear to have skin test conversion following repeated testing--a result of the "booster effect". In short, the tuberculin skin test may be of limited diagnostic usefulness in the evaluation of findings in the individual patient. Bacteriology remains the cornerstone of diagnosis.

CULTURES FOR MYCOBACTERIA

The probability of recovering mycobacteria in cultures is directly related to the quality of the material being cultured. Negative mycobacterial cultures obtained from spontaneous sputum specimens from patients with a nonproductive or minimal cough usually signify only the lack of mycobacteria in the saliva of the individual patient. If one hopes to recover mycobacteria, an adequate specimen must be obtained.

SPUTUM

The greatest opportunity for recovering mycobacteria from the sputum occurs with an early morning collection, when the patient has pooled tracheobronchial secretions. This is true in those who are able to spontaneously produce an adequate sputum specimen and is even more important in the patient who requires induction of cough and expectoration. The use of aerosols containing normal saline, water, and 10 percent sodium chloride and glycerin, to produce expectoration, are all adequate methods of obtaining sputum specimens. Ultrasonic water aerosol is also effective for many patients. It has been shown that the use of routine gastric washings for mycobacterial culture following collection of a postinduction sputum specimen enhances diagnostic capability.[2] Even in the presence of the above methods of sputum induction, some patients will still be unable to produce an adequate sputum specimen. Adequate culture specimens must be obtained by other means in such patients. In selected cases, one may consider transtracheal aspiration, bronchoscopy with bronchial washings and brushings, and even transbronchoscopic lung biopsy. The decision to use these more aggressive invasive techniques will depend largely on the clinical situation.

GASTRIC WASHINGS

Gastric washings remain an excellent method of obtaining culture specimens in the patient who is unable to expectorate adequate material. Gastric washings are also ideally obtained early in the morning in the fasting patient when material, brought up during the night by the mucociliary clearance mechanism and spontaneously swallowed, is pooled in the stomach. Lavage of the stomach with sterile saline after removing the pooled gastric contents may improve the quality and volume of the specimen.

At this point, we should mention the use of acid-fast stains in the evaluation of gastric aspiration specimens. As a rule, we do not stain these gastric specimens for acid-fast bacilli (AFB) as positive stains for AFB will frequently confuse the situation. A large percentage of normal persons harbor nonpathogenic, saprophytic acid-fast organisms in the stomach contents, but their presence is not necessarily diagnostic of an *M. tuberculosis* infection. This is also true of urine specimens.

PLEURAL FLUID

The staining and culture of pleural fluid for mycobacteria remains worthwhile, although the yield of positive results is low in patients with documented tuberculous pleuritis. Needle biopsy of the pleura with appropriate culture techniques produces a much higher yield of positive mycobacterial cultures and concomitant tissue sections stained with H & E and, for AFB, may confirm the pathologic process.[3]

URINE

Cultures obtained from a midstream first morning urine specimen give the highest yield of positive cultures for mycobacteria. Twelve- and twenty-four-hour urine specimens tend to become contaminated with bacteria, especially gram negative organisms, which make subsequent contamination and overgrowth of the culture material a significant problem.

TISSUE ASPIRATES AND BODY FLUIDS

Lymph nodes, peritoneum, joints, epididymis, pericardium and even lung may be aspirated, under appropriate circumstances, for AFB stains and culture.

BIOPSY

Needle biopsy of the pleura, liver, bone, synovium, peritoneum, pericardium, bone marrow and lung, may be necessary to establish the diagnosis of tuberculosis in certain circumstances. Techniques of fiberoptic transbronchoscopic biopsy, brushing and washing have reduced the indications for transthoracic needle biopsy of the lung for diagnosis. In certain cases, all attempts short of some type of open surgical biopsy fail, and confirmation can only be made in this manner.

LABORATORY METHODS

A discussion of the techniques currently used to stain, isolate and identify mycobacteria is beyond the scope of this monograph. Briefly, most specimens are digested and decontaminated to kill rapidly growing contaminating organisms and to liquify organic debris. The specimen is then inoculated onto suitable media and incubated for up to eight weeks. Mycobacteria will usually be isolated within three to six weeks. Smears of the specimen are also stained for acid-fast bacilli, using one of the conventional methods such as Ziehl-Neelsen or Kinyon stain. Newer techniques of staining, using the fluorochrome procedure with stains such as auramine and rhodamine, are much more sensitive and have become widely used for screening specimens. Specimens which are positive with the fluorochrome procedure should be double-checked with a conventional stain such as Ziehl-Neelsen, as false-positive results are common. Overinterpretation of fluorochrome stains has become a definite problem in the hands of less experienced laboratories. As a general rule, gastric aspirates and urine specimens should not be stained for AFB, as a positive result cannot be interpreted due to the high incidence of saprophytic acid-fast organisms.

A more detailed description of methods used to process clinical specimens for mycobacteria can be obtained by reading one of several excellent references describing these laboratory methods.[4, 5]

CASE REPORT

The following case history exemplifies some of the problems that may be encountered in evaluating the findings in a patient suspected of having tuberculosis.

A 50-year-old woman was admitted to the hospital in May, 1975, with a two-week history of pleuritic pain in the right side of the chest, low-grade fever and nonproductive cough. Results of the physical examination were consistent with a right pleural effusion, but were otherwise unremarkable. The admission laboratory studies were unremarkable. The chest roentgenogram (Fig. 2. 1) revealed a large, right pleural effusion.

Induced sputa followed by gastric washings were obtained on three consecutive days. The AFB stains on the gastric washings were positive. However, the sputum AFB stains were negtive. An intermediate PPD skin test was negative. The pleural fluid was consistent with an exudate and pleural fluid AFB stains were negative. The pleural fluid cytology was also negative. A Cope needle biopsy of the parietal pleura revealed noncaseating granuloma. No AFB were seen on special stains of the pleura. The initial positive gastric washing AFB stains had prompted the physician to institute antituberculous chemotherapy. However, the subsequent combination of the finding of AFB-negative noncaseating granuloma in the pleural biopsy specimen, in combination with a negative PPD skin test, led him to change his diagnosis to sarcoidosis. He then elected to discontinue the antituberculous therapy and start treatment with corticosteroids.

We first saw the patient at this time. She was understandably perplexed because she was told that she had tuberculosis (because of a positive gastric AFB stain), then told she did not have TB (negative PPD and noncaseating granulomas on pleural biopsy). Our diagnostic evaluation consisted of repeating the studies of the pleural fluid and needle biopsy of the pleura. The pleural fluid and pleural biopsy were again negative on AFB stain. The tissue specimens again revealed noncaseating granulomas. At this time, the cultures of both the sputum and gastric washings from the other hospital were negative, after six weeks, for M. tuberculosis. The gastric washings had grown M. aquae, Runyon group 2 scotochromogens, which are frequently recovered from gastric washings. A PPD (5 TU) skin test was positive, and we elected to reestablish antituberculous

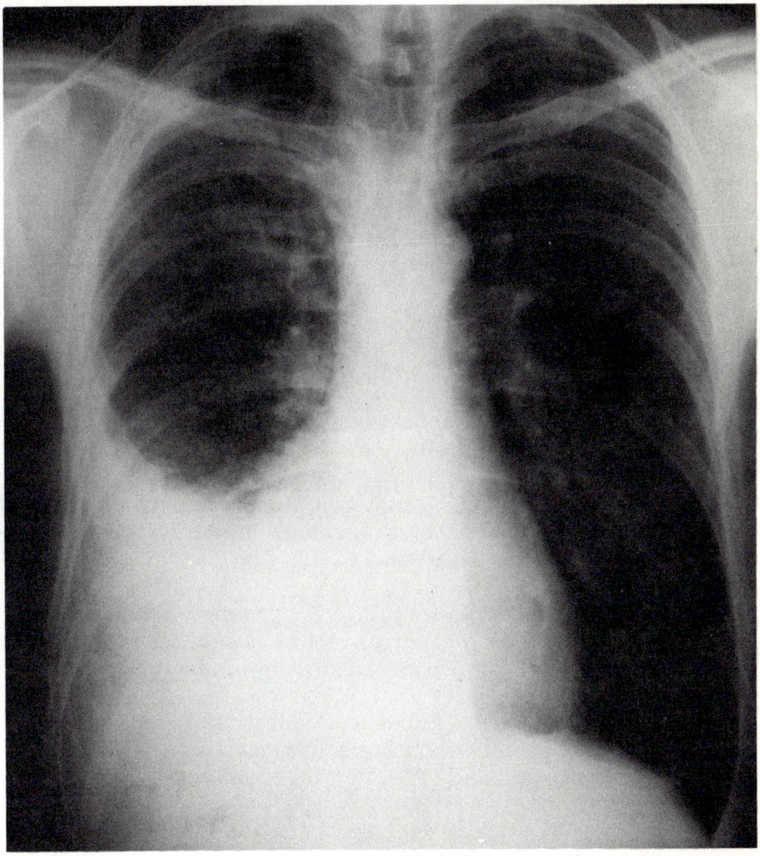

FIG. 2.1: Large right pleural effusion resulting from tuberculous pleuritis with effusion.

chemotherapy while awaiting the results of our pleural fluid and pleural tissue mycobacterial cultures. Subsequently, the pleural tissue cultures were positive for M. tuberculosis. Pleural fluid cultures were negative. The patient had a prompt clinical and radiologic response to chemotherapy and the pleural effusion cleared completely within ten weeks.

This case illustrates the hazards of misinterpreting positive gastric AFB smears and the results of the PPD skin tests. It also illustrates the value of pleural tissue cultures in tuberculous pleuritis. In addition, the interpretation of noncaseating granulomas as synonymous with sarcoidosis is a common pitfall. Although sarcoid pleural effusion may rarely be seen, this is a diagnosis of exclusion. In the final analysis, tuberculosis is also a diagnosis of exclusion in the patient described and can only be excluded by obtaining adequate and appropriate culture material.

REFERENCES

1. Youmans GP: Relation between delayed hypersensitivity and immunity in tuberculosis. Am Rev Respir Dis 111:109, 1975.

2. Carr DT, Karlson AG, et al.: A comparison of cultures of induced sputum and gastric washings in the diagnosis of tuberculosis. Mayo Clin Proc 42:23, 1967.

3. Levine H, Metzger W, et al.: Diagnosis of tuberculous pleurisy by culture of pleural biopsy specimen. Arch Intern Med 126:269, 1970.

4. Kubica GP, Dye WE: Laboratory methods for clinical and public health mycobacteriology. Atlanta, Department of Health, Education and Welfare, US, 1967.

5. Vestal AL: Procedures for the isolation and identification of mycobacteria. Atlanta, Department of Health, Education and Welfare, US, 1975.

CHAPTER III:

TUBERCULIN SKIN TESTING AND PREVENTIVE THERAPY

TUBERCULIN SKIN TESTING

The standard technique for tuberculin skin testing (Mantoux) utilizes purified protein derivative (PPD) tuberculin, stabilized with Tween 80 and standardized by biologic assay to 5 tuberculin units.[1] The antigen (0. 1 mg) is injected intracutaneously into the skin on the volar or dorsal surface of the forearm using a one-half inch . 26 or . 27-gauge needle. A discrete wheal 6 to 10 mm in diameter should be produced if the test is applied properly. The antigen should be drawn into the syringe and used immediately to avoid absorption onto the plastic or glass surface of the syringe. The reaction should then be recorded at forty-eight or seventy-two hours in terms of induration transverse to the long axis of the forearm. Erythema without evidence of induration is not considered significant. If, however, the antigen is inappropriately injected subcutaneously, erythema may occur with equivocal or no induration, and the test should be repeated.

A positive Mantoux Test reaction is obtained if the diameter of induration is 10 mm or more. Induration of from 5 to 9 mm constitutes a doubtful reaction and should be repeated. Less than 4 mm induration at forty-eight and seventy-two hours is a negative reaction and need not be repeated. As noted, only induration of 10 mm or more is considered a positive reaction. However, reactions in the doubtful range in subjects in close contact with patients with active tuberculosis (Group 1), must be considered potentially positive and repeated in three months. In practice, many physicians consider induration of 9 mm or more to be a positive reaction.

Multiple puncture tuberculin tests such as the tine and mono-vacc. tests are widely used for routine screening, especially by pediatricians. There is no way to standardize the amount of antigen injected with these multiple-puncture techniques and they are frequently difficult to interpret. Although specific recommendations are given regarding the interpretation of the multiple puncture test (i. e. less than 2 mm induration is negative), we feel that should any degree of induration develop, a repeat test utilizing the standard Mantoux reaction is indicated.

CANDIDATES FOR PREVENTIVE THERAPY

It appears to us, from our contact with practicing physicians, that nothing in the area of tuberculosis management has been more confusing than the concept of preventive therapy. Changes in the recommendations for preventive chemotherapy, the widely reported severe or sometimes fatal reactions in patients receiving preventive therapy with isoniazid (INH), and the disagreement among "experts" on the indications for preventive therapy have perpetuated this state of confusion.

The initial enthusiasm for preventive chemotherapy of tuberculosis with INH was dampened by subsequent reports of serious and fatal cases of INH-associated hepatitis. The current guidelines for the use of preventive therapy of tuberculosis were adopted by a joint committee of the American Thoracic Society, American Lung Association and the Center for Disease Control. [2]

At present, the efficacy of INH in the prevention of progressive infection in the group of patients with positive reactions to tuberculin skin tests, but without evidence of active disease, appears to be well documented. [3]

The patient with a positive skin test and a normal chest roentgenogram or Ranke complex with a Ghon lesion is felt to benefit from preventive drug therapy by a reduction in the residual mycobacterial population remaining in "healed" lesions and roentgenographically invisible residual lesions. This eradication or reduction of residual bacteria decreases the incidence of reactivation and progressive disease later in the patient's life. In considering the individual patient for preventive chemotherapy, we must weigh the potential benefit of INH therapy against the potential for adverse reaction to the drug during the course of therapy. The major adverse reaction to INH is INH-associated hepatitis. Current recommendations for preventive therapy with INH include selection of a group of high-risk, priority patients in whom the chance of developing progressive tuberculosis far outweighs the risk of adverse reaction to INH. [2] These groups are:

(1) household members and other close associates of

persons with a recent diagnosis of active tuberculous disease

(2) positive tuberculin skin test reactors, with findings on the chest roentgenogram consistent with nonprogressive tuberculous disease, in whom there are neither positive bacteriologic findings nor a history of adequate chemotherapy

(3) newly infected persons (recent skin test converters)

(4) positive tuberculin skin test reactors in special clinical situations

(5) other positive skin test reactors.

We will discuss each of these groups individually. Each group presents a different type of problem, since the risk of developing progressive disease within the period of the patient's anticipated life expectancy and the risk of serious adverse reaction to INH varies with each patient. In general, the risk of progressive tuberculosis is greatest in infancy, adolescence and early adult life. This risk, however, continues throughout life in all patients with a positive tuberculin skin test. Data suggest that the degree of risk can be directly related to the degree of positivity of the skin test reaction.[4] In addition, patients who are skin-test positive, bacteriologically negative and have significant residual changes on the chest roentgenogram are also much more likely to develop subsequent progressive infection. Conversely, the risk of serious, adverse reaction to INH is minimal in younger patients, increasing significantly after the age of 35 to 45 years.[4, 5] All of these factors must be considered in making a decision regarding preventive therapy with INH in the individual patient.

Group 1 may fall into two general categories, according to age. These subjects, all contacts of a patient with recently confirmed active tuberculosis, may be children with known previous negative skin tests or without any prior tuberculin tests who remain negative when tested or are now positive. Most authorities would suggest that these children with negative skin tests, who are in close contact with a patient with a recent diagnosis of tuberculosis, be placed on INH therapy. Children with a skin test that is positive or doubtful, (induration of 5 mm or more with a 5 TU intradermal skin test), should receive INH for one year if roentgenographically negative. Positive chest roentgenograms should be followed with bacteriologic evaluation for progressive disease. Children with negative skin tests should be placed on INH therapy, as they may be infected and not yet have converted the skin test. If, on repeat testing in three months, the child's skin test remains negative and exposure has ended, the INH therapy may be discontinued. We would continue treating the child with a doubtful positive (5 to 9 mm induration) skin test with INH for one year. Conversion of the skin test to positive after three months is an indication for continuation of the INH for a total of twelve months.

The problem with the adults in Group 1 is a little more difficult. The adult contact may have a negative skin test, and in this situation the age of the contact (potential risk of adverse INH reaction) and the degree of infectiousness of the patient with active disease must be considered. As a general rule, we have not given INH to contacts over 35 years of age with negative skin tests and have elected to repeat the tuberculin test at four and twelve weeks. If the adult contact's skin test has converted, he is placed on a 12-month course of INH. If the skin test is still negative after three months and the exposure has ended, we suggest that the contact be followed with an annual tuberculin skin test. The contact who is already skin-test positive is handled in the manner outlined for patients in Group 5.

Patients with positive tuberculin skin tests and abnormal chest roentgenograms (Group 2) may be previous tuberculosis patients who have had either no chemotherapy or inadequate chemotherapy, or newly discovered but inactive tuberculosis. These patients should have complete bacteriologic evaluation to rule out bacteriologically positive and progressive disease. If bacteriologic studies are negative, INH chemotherapy should be instituted for a total of twelve months. The rate of reactivation in this group of patients with positive skin tests and abnormal chest roentgenograms has been variously reported to range from one to five percent per year. Most of these patients are over 40 years of age and at increased risks for adverse reactions to INH. However, the risk of developing progressive disease appears to outweigh the risk of INH hepatitis, especially if the patient is observed closely for clinical symptoms and liver function changes (enzymes) of INH hepatitis.

Newly infected patients (Group 3) are those who have developed a positive tuberculin skin test and have had a documented negative skin test within the prior two years. This group is extremely important because it is felt that the more recent the tuberculosis infection, the greater the chance of developing progressive disease. It is estimated that five percent of newly infected patients develop progressive tuberculosis within the first year after infection. When dealing with children, this category of skin test reactor is frequently a rather straightforward problem because a large number of children are tested annually by private physicians and in school programs. The problem arises in older patients who have supposedly converted the tuberculin skin test. Variations in technique of application and ability to interpret skin tests must be considered a possible cause of prior skin-test negativity and unless the same physician has done the prior skin testing, one can never be sure that it was negative. This is an important consideration since, as stated previously, the incidence of serious adverse INH reactions is more common in this older group of patients. In addition, one must consider two other causes for "false skin-test conversion." The first is the phenomenon of the "booster effect" seen in older patients when two tuberculosis skin tests are placed within a short period of time. In this situation, an older patient with tuberculosis exposure and limited infection years before may well have a doubtful positive skin test for tuberculin. However, if he is retested in the next year he may be found to have a definite positive test. This is frequently not a conversion from negative to positive but reflects a boost in the delayed hypersensitivity reaction that the renewed experience with tuberculin antigen from the prior skin test produced. This "booster effect" is extremely rare in persons under the age of 50 years, but must be kept in mind as a potential reason for an apparent skin test conversion in the older patient.

The other cause of a false-positive skin test conversion is a recent blood transfusion. Patients with negative tuberculin skin tests may convert to positive shortly after receiving a blood transfusion from a tuberculin-positive donor. This positive skin test is of limited duration, but must be kept in mind when apparent tuberculin test conversion is noted in the older patient.

Group 4 includes patients who are candidates for INH preventive therapy who have a positive tuberculin test and are felt to be at significantly greater risk of developing progressive tuberculosis. The tuberculin-positive subject with prolonged corticosteroid treatment, for any reason other than normal adrenocortical replacement, should receive INH therapy. Whether INH should be given to these patients as long as they are on steroids, or for one year, remains a matter of controversy. Additional indications for one-year preventive therapy with INH include: immunosuppresive therapy, certain hematologic and reticuloendothelial diseases such as Hodgkin's disease and leukemia, diabetes mellitus, silicosis and gastrectomy. The use of preventive INH in the tuberculin-negative anergic or immunosuppressed patient receiving therapeutic corticosteroids is a controversial subject. We tend to use INH in this situation. The relationship of progressive tuberculosis to gastrectomy is also controversial. However, at this time it is recommended that these patients receive INH for one year if the tuberculin skin test is positive.

Most of the controversy regarding preventive INH therapy has revolved around the last group of patients (Group 5). These are the positive tuberculin skin test reactors who do not fall into the other four groups. On the whole, these are patients who have positive tuberculin skin tests without ever having a skin test before--those who have had a negative skin test well over two years previously or just cannot recall if they have ever been skin tested or, if they have, the result. The decision as to whether or not to give these patients INH is made on the basis of age. If the subject is less than 35 years of age, the risk of developing progressive tuberculosis during his lifetime appears to outweigh the risk of INH hepatitis during the year of INH therapy. Certainly, all bacteriologically negative tuberculin skin test reactors under the age of 35 years should receive a year of INH preventive therapy. INH treatment is felt to be mandatory in children, especially those below the age of 7 years.[2] A recent editorial by Comstock and Edwards[5] suggests that the upper age limit for INH preventive therapy could have been set at 45 years of age without additional risk factors.

CONTACT EVALUATION

Evaluation of individuals exposed to the patient with active tuberculosis and treatment of skin test converters is an important aspect of preventive therapy. A logical approach to the evaluation of contacts for infection requires a detailed family, social, and occupational assessment of the patient. A practical, economical, and yet useful contact evaluation involves some method between no evaluation and skin testing of everyone who knows the patient. In addition, there are social and economic implications for the individual patient when large numbers of low-risk contacts are subjected to skin test evaluation. Indiscriminate contact evaluation may be nonproductive and may even cause the patient embarrassment and loss of employment.

The most important factors in evaluating the infectiousness of the patient with active tuberculosis are sputum-smear positivity, proximity of exposure, and duration of exposure. The sputum-smear negative patient is seldom infectious. On the other hand, the smear-positive patient with laryngeal tuberculosis may infect scores of people.

At the present time, the "Concentric Circle" approach to contact evaluation appears to be the most logical method for evaluating contacts for infection. This method involves the sequential and systematic skin testing of contacts on the basis of the degree of exposure. The most heavily exposed group would, in most instances, be the patient's immediate family which constitutes the "first circle". If all family members are skin-test negative, it is unlikely that less intimately exposed contacts would be infected and no further contact evaluation would be warranted. However, if one or two of the patient's children, for example, were skin-test positive, further contact evaluation would be indicated and we would move on to the "second circle". The "second circle" would involve occupational contacts if the patient works outside of the home or close social contacts. A weekly bridge group might be evaluated in the case of an unemployed housewife who is found to have skin-test positive children. If contacts in the "second circle" were found to be recent skin test converters, the next circle would include more casual contacts. This "Concentric Circle" approach, when used properly, leads to appropriate contact evaluation.

It may be necessary to segregate contacts at the occupational level into several circles based on proximity and duration of contact. If, for example, the patient works in an office with ten employees but within a company with hundreds of employees, the ten employees most intimately associated would constitute the "second circle". If the employees in this "second circle" were not infected, no further evaluation would be indicated at the patient's place of employment. As noted before, if the "first circle" contacts are not infected, we would proceed no further.

EVALUATION OF INDIVIDUAL CANDIDATES FOR INH PREVENTIVE THERAPY

Once the individual patient is placed in one of the previously mentioned categories, further evaluation is required to ascertain that he is a candidate for twelve months of INH therapy. The first step is to obtain a chest roentgenogram to rule out active or progressive tuberculosis. If the chest roentgenogram suggests the possibility of active diseases, complete medical and bacteriologic evaluation is imperative. Many patients are seen with parenchymal changes interpreted as "old inactive tuberculosis", and a significant number of these patients will have bacteriologically positive findings. Comparison of current and previous chest roentgenograms may reveal slow progression of the infiltrate but, even in the presence of an apparently stable lesion, bacteriologic evaluation should be carried out if significant parenchymal changes are present. INH therapy alone is inadequate treatment in the bacteriologically positive patient and this possibility must be evaluated in all patients with a positive chest roentgenogram.

A history of adequate INH therapy may be obtained from some patients and this possibility must be evaluated. In addition, a history of experience with INH resulting in adverse reactions such as INH-associated hepatic injury, drug fever, arthritis, CNS symptoms and nonspecific reactions such as chills, fever and myalgia is a contraindication to further INH therapy.

Acute liver disease of any etiology is a contraindication to preventive INH therapy as is chronic liver disease in most situations. Chronic alcohol abuse may be associated with a higher incidence of INH hepatitis and chronic alcohol consumption with liver enzyme abnormalities frequently makes the evaluation for INH-associated hepatitis extremely difficult. In addition, the alcholic patient is frequently too unreliable to assure adequate follow-up for adverse reactions to INH. Chronic alcoholism alone is not an absolute contraindication to INH therapy, however.

The chronic use of other medications which may interact with INH must be considered. An example is diphenylhydantoin, which may be excreted at a decreased rate in the presence of INH, leading to diphenylhydantoin toxicity.

For medicolegal reasons, it is recommended that INH not be given as preventive therapy during pregnancy. INH has not been shown to be harmful to the fetus, but it is recommended that preventive INH therapy be started after delivery during the period of greatest risk of tuberculosis in the mother. We would stress that this discussion of the relative contraindications for INH apply to preventive therapy and that the use of INH, in addition to other drugs, in active disease with close monitoring is acceptable in certain clinical situations, such as pregnancy.

PATIENT FOLLOW-UP DURING PREVENTIVE INH TREATMENT PROGRAM

Once the decision is made to commence a twelve-month

course of preventive therapy with INH, the physician has two charges. First, the patient must be well informed as to the natural history of tuberculosis and the rationale for preventive therapy with INH. The patient must understand the reason for daily medication for twelve months, despite the fact that he feels well. Secondly, the patient must also be made aware of the signs and symptoms of adverse INH reactions. He is instructed to contact his physician promptly if he notes unexplained fever, malaise, nausea, vomiting or myalgia. Persistent paresthesias and dermatitis may also signify an adverse reaction to INH and require prompt evaluation. Advanced hepatic injury may rarely occur in the absence of systemic symptoms and the patient must immediately report the occurrence of dark urine, icterus or generalized pruritus.

Routine monitoring of all patients receiving preventive INH with serum glutamic oxaloacetic transaminase (SGOT) determination is an extremely controversial topic. It has been suggested that routine SGOT monitoring is not necessary and that monthly questioning of the patient in regard to symptoms of toxicity will suffice.[2] If the patient has symptoms of toxicity, the SGOT level is checked. Some physicians feel that the patient on preventive treatment should have an SGOT level determination at one, two, three, six and nine months while on INH. Many patients, especially those who use alcohol regularly, may show mild elevation of SGOT levels while on INH therapy. If the SGOT value does not exceed three times normal and no signs or symptoms of INH toxicity are present, the elevation of the SGOT level *per se* is not an indication for discontinuing therapy. If the SGOT value is elevated to more than three times the upper limit of normal, the INH should be discontinued and not reinstituted. As stated previously, the incidence of INH-associated liver enzyme abnormalities increases with age and is rare in children.

The recommended dose of INH is 300 mg once daily for adults and 10 mg/kg/body weight/day, not to exceed 300 mg for children. The routine use of pyridoxine in this dosage range is not mandatory but may be advisable.

BCG VACCINATION

BCG vaccination has been reported to produce highly variable results in the prevention of progressive tuberculosis. The results of BCG vaccination in preventing active tuberculosis in some studies carried out in underdeveloped and urban areas with very high rates of infection, have been reported to be excellent. On the other hand, studies by the U.S. Public Health

Service have failed to show a significant reduction in the case rate of tuberculosis in controlled studies. There are many theories regarding the discrepancies between the results of these various studies of BCG; poor statistical methods and program design, prior infection with atypical mycobacteria and variations in BCG potency have all been blamed for the rather poor results obtained.

Although BCG vaccinations may be a reasonable alternative in underdeveloped areas with limited resources, it would appear that the uncertain efficacy of BCG and the availability of isoniazid makes BCG less desirable for use in highly developed areas, with certain exceptions. One of the criticisms of BCG vaccination is the fact that it converts the PPD skin test, making it useless in screening for patients with M. tuberculosis. At present, it would appear that a well-conducted program of INH preventive therapy in skin test converters has distinct advantages over BCG vaccination in highly developed countries such as the United States. However, this remains a highly controversial subject.

In summary, the eventual eradication of tuberculosis will require more than a search for patients with symptoms or roentgenographic signs of active tuberculosis. A comprehensive program which will locate subjects with positive reactions to tuberculin skin tests, especially recent converters, with no evidence of active or progressive disease, and establish an adequate period of preventive INH therapy is essential if tuberculosis is to be conquered. The problems attending selection of candidates for preventive INH therapy are slowly resolving, but the challenge of the reservoir of positive skin test reactors (Group 5) above the age of 35 to 45 years remains. Weighing the statistical benefit of the prevention of progressive tuberculosis against the projected incidence of INH-associated hepatitis, it appears that annual chest roentgenographic follow-up is the best answer to this problem at present.

We have not discussed the more unusual problems in preventive therapy such as the prophylactic treatment of the contact exposed to infectious tuberculous patients with significant drug-resistant disease. This has not been considered a significant problem in the United States, but may become more common. Immigration of patients with drug-resistant progressive tuberculosis from the Orient has become a significant problem in military dependents, especially those from Korea and Japan. Recent data suggest that in situations where the major drug resistance is suspected, preventive INH therapy of close tuberculous contacts may be ineffective and that rifampin may be a more effective preventive agent.[8] Since a controlled study has not been performed, such reports must be considered anecdotal. In those situations where significant drug resistance is known or suspected, early consultation with an expert in the chemotherapy of tuberculosis is imperative for the adequate management of both the patient and close contacts.

REFERENCES

1. American Lung Association: Diagnostic Standards and Classification of Tuberculosis and Other Mycobacterial Diseases. New York, American Lung Association, 1974.

2. American Thoracic Society: Preventive therapy of tuberculous infection. Am Rev Respir Dis 110:371, 1974.

3. Comstock GW, Woolpert SF, et al.: Isoniazid prophylaxis among Alaskan Eskimos. A progress report. Am Rev Respir Dis 110:195, 1974.

4. Doto IL, Furcolow ML, et al.: Size of the tuberculin reaction. Relationship to subsequent development of tuberculosis in Kansas - Missouri area. Arch Environ Health 23: 392, 1971.

5. Edwards PQ: Isoniazid-associated hepatitis. (Abstract) Am Rev Respir Dis 109:717, 1974.

6. Comstock GW, Edwards PQ: The competing risks of tuberculosis and hepatitis for adult tuberculin reactors. Am Rev Respir Dis 111:573, 1975.

7. Comstock GW, Livesay VT, et al.: Evaluation of BCG vaccination among Puerto Rican children. Am J Public Health 64:283, 1974.

8. Fairshter RD, Randazzo GP, et al.: Failure of isoniazid prophylaxis after exposure to isoniazid-resistant tuberculosis. Am Rev Respir Dis 112:37, 1975.

CHAPTER IV:

THE TREATMENT OF TUBERCULOSIS

PRINCIPLES OF CHEMOTHERAPY

The successful treatment of a patient infected with Mycobacterium tuberculosis requires knowledge of the following: the nature of the infecting organism; an estimate of the number of organisms within the patient; the mechanism of action and side effects of the drugs available for treatment; and familiarity with the patient's life style and the resources available in the community.

NATURE OF THE INFECTING ORGANISM

Isoniazid resistance occurs naturally in 1 out of 100,000 tuberculous organisms and streptomycin resistance occurs in about 1 organism per 1,000,000 bacilli. Drug resistance will almost invariably develop if only one drug is used when larger populations of bacilli are present, because resistant mutants develop with predictable frequency in the presence or absence of a drug.[1] Hence, resistant mutants may be present in the patient prior to the initiation of therapy. If, for example, 100,000,000 bacilli are present in a patient with cavitary disease, many resistant mutants could be expected. However, these mutants are resistant to a single drug and double drug resistance and cross-resistance usually are not found in patients who have not received prior drug therapy. Thus, when a patient with tuberculosis receives two drugs to which the infecting organism is susceptible, those bacilli resistant to the first drug would be killed by the second; and similarly, those resistant to the second drug would be killed by the first.

NUMBER OF ORGANISMS WITHIN THE PATIENT

Canetti has shown that the bacillary population of a tuberculous lesion varies according to its morphology.[2] The greatest number of organisms are found in cavity walls where 100,000,000 organisms may be present in contrast to nodular pulmonary lesions which contain about 1,000 bacilli. The patient with a positive PPD skin test who does not have roentgenographically demonstrable pulmonary disease, has even fewer bacilli-perhaps 100 organisms or less. Therefore, bacteriologically positive patients with extensive cavitary pulmonary disease harbor very large populations of organisms while in patients with other forms of pulmonary and extrapulmonary tuberculosis the number of bacilli present is much smaller.

The number of organisms remaining in the patient after drug therapy has been instituted also must be considered. This estimate determines the necessity for and duration of intensive multiple drug therapy and the total duration of therapy. After the early phase of drug therapy, usually three to six months, has reduced the bacterial population to 10, 000 organisms or less, the possibility of developing resistant mutants becomes very unlikely. At this point, less intensive drug therapy is required and the number of drugs may be reduced if more than two drugs are being used. The total duration of chemotherapy and the need for prolonged therapy currently are under investigation. Nevertheless, if the initial period of therapy is accomplished without problems and the sputum bacteriology becomes smear and culture negative within three to six months and remain negative, a total duration of therapy of eighteen to twenty-four months would be conservative and, while perhaps longer than absolutely necessary, would ensure a successful outcome. Continuing isoniazid alone for a more prolonged period, even a lifetime, in those patients with persistent extensive roentgenographic abnormalities is not justified.

DRUG ACTIONS AND SIDE EFFECTS

Antituberculous drugs are effective because they disrupt various metabolic processes of the tuberculosis organisms. The principle site of action of isoniazid is in DNA synthesis while ethambutol and rifampin effect RNA and streptomycin protein synthesis. Bacteriocidal drugs are more effective than bacteriostatic drugs, the latter by necessity having to rely partially upon the immune system of the host. Isoniazid, rifampin, streptomycin and the other aminoglycoside drugs, and ethionamide are bacteriocidal drugs, while ethambutol, para-aminosalicyclic acid (PAS) pyrazinamide, and cycloserine are bacteriostatic drugs.

Antituberculous drugs may produce side effects varying from unimportant to life threatening. Table II (Appendix 2) lists the side effects, dose and characteristics of the antituberculous drugs used in the United States. Each of the side effects of the drugs that may be prescribed for a patient must be known, as well as whether it is necessary to monitor for such side effects.

Isoniazid has been associated with a number of central nervous system symptoms such as dizziness, muscular twitching and, rarely, convulsions. Such central nervous system side effects due to isoniazid are rare and cease after discontinuing the drug. Not uncommon is a feeling of excitement and hyperactivity if the entire 300 mg of isoniazid is taken at one time and usually follows approximately eight hours after ingestion. This is alleviated by dividing the dose throughout the day. The advantage of administering the entire dose once a day is better patient compliance. Pyridoxine hydrochloride prevents the peripheral neuritis that has been observed following isoniazid therapy, and while probably unnecessary in most patients, it is recommended that all patients, including children who receive isoniazid, also take pyridoxine. Very rarely are there hypersensitivity reactions to isoniazid which include fever, rash and a lupus-like picture.

By far the most important side effect of isoniazid is the liver disease that has been associated with isoniazid therapy. The clinical features of isoniazid-induced liver disease are clinically, biochemically and histologically indistinguishable from viral hepatitis.[3] In mild cases, histologic examination of the liver has demonstrated focal areas of hepatocellular necrosis. In more severe cases, the syndrome resembles typical viral hepatitis and begins with malaise, anorexia and nausea, with or without vomiting, before the development of jaundice. Some patients may complain initially of a viral-like illness while others are completely asymptomatic until the onset of jaundice. Biochemical tests yield the pattern of acute hepatocellular necrosis with high transaminase and moderately elevated alkaline phosphatase values. A minority of patients demonstrate a mixed pattern of hepatocellular and cholestatic jaundice. The histologic pattern characteristic of viral hepatitis is seen with extensive bridging and fibrosis suggesting that chronic irreversible liver damage may occur.

Mild or more severe liver injury may occur from one week to many months after the initiation of isoniazid therapy; however, the majority of cases of isoniazid-associated hepatitis occur within the first three months of treatment. In most patients improvement occurs shortly after isoniazid has been discontinued and is almost always complete. Monitoring liver enzymes has not proven to be useful in detecting isoniazid-associated hepatitis except in those patients who report gastrointestinal symptoms such as anorexia, nausea, vomiting or jaundice. It is essential that the patient understand fully the potential toxic side effects and be instructed to both discontinue his isoniazid and to seek medical care when such symptoms occur. Prompt cessation of the drug causes a return toward normal of the bilirubin and enzymes. Indeed, a rapid improvement of liver function tests is often more characteristic of drug-associated hepatitis than of viral hepatitis or alcoholic liver disease.

Both isoniazid and rifampin have been demonstrated to participate in important drug interactions. Isoniazid has been shown to interfere with the metabolism of dilantin and patients receiving both isoniazid and dilantin should be instructed about the potential for, and observed for, dilantin overdosage. In such patients, the dilantin dose should be lowered while receiving isoniazid and the dilantin dose increased after the isoniazid has been discontinued. Rifampin has been shown to be a potent inducer of drug metabolism, as it causes a proliferation of the smooth endoplasmic reticulum and an increase of cytochrome P450 content in the liver.[4] It also increases its own rate of desacetylation. There is a selectivity in the enzyme induction effect of rifampin for anticoagulants such as warfarin sodium, oral hypoglycemic agents, corticosteroids, methadone and oral contraceptives. Pregnancy has occurred in women receiving oral contraceptives, withdrawal has been experienced in patients on methadone maintenance and warfarin sodium requirements for anticoagulation have increased in patients also receiving rifampin. Conversely, these effects are reversed after the discontinuation of rifampin; overcoagulation, for example, has occurred following the discontinuation of rifampin in patients maintained on warfarin sodium.

A flu-like syndrome may be produced by rifampin. Also the patient's urine, tears and saliva may turn orange following the initiation of rifampin and this requires only patient reassurance and not discontinuation of the drug. However, more serious side effects of rifampin include renal failure, hemolysis and thrombocytopenia. The thrombocytopenia results from the absorption of antirifampin antibodies onto platelets which, after fixing complement, result in platelet damage. Such reactions require immediate discontinuation of rifampin. Rifampin associated hepatitis is similar to that observed following administration of isoniazid and should be watched for with careful instruction of the patient and prompt discontinuation of the drug at the onset of suspicious symptoms. As with isoniazid, routine monitoring of liver function tests is not fruitful. The liver toxicity of isoniazid and rifampin appears to be additive, not synergistic, and does not necessarily preclude the administration of either or both drugs to alcoholic patients with or without liver disease. However, considerable caution should be exercised in the care of patients with pre-existent liver disease and efforts to limit the number of potentially hepatotoxic drugs given are warranted.

Streptomycin has long been known to be nephrotoxic and to cause eighth cranial nerve damage. It should be used with caution in the presence of renal insufficiency. Audiograms, tests of vestibular function and renal function, are indicated as a base-line and later if symptoms occur. Neuromuscular junction blockade has rarely been observed in patients receiving both streptomycin and muscle relaxants or with pre-existing myasthenia gravis. Hypersensitivity reactions such as rash and dermatitis may also occur. Streptomycin should be discontinued in such patients.

The use of ethambutol requires base-line visual acuity and red-green color discrimination tests but no further monitoring is necessary in the absence of eye symptoms if a dose of 15 mg/kg/day is being used. Routine monitoring is indicated if the dose is 25 mg/kg/day. The gastrointestinal side effects of PAS are so frequent that PAS is no longer used as a primary drug in adults. Children appear to tolerate PAS much better than adults although hypersensitivity reactions such as fever, rash and arthritis have been reported.

PATIENT'S LIFE STYLE AND COMMUNITY RESOURCES

Organizing an effective ambulatory care facility is the most important and often most challenging problem that must be solved in caring for patients with tuberculosis. Whether one is involved in a large program in an urban ghetto or in a rural setting with a few patients, the basic issue is patient compliance. The only meaningful measure of success is the percentage of patients who complete therapy.

An approach must be fashioned around the specific needs of the patient population. For example, a skid-row population will require the availability of social services and a clinic staff that can relate humanely to patients who are alcoholics. The working patient and family member may need more assistance in advocacy and in educating the employer and community to accept them. Staff must be able and willing to diplomatically accomplish these tasks.

The difficulty in determining which patient will be compliant makes it necessary to approach every patient as potentially noncompliant. A punitive or parenteral approach has been proven to be ineffective. Rather, the approach should be to work with the patient in removing as many barriers to compliance, as possible. The patient should have a clear understanding of his role in curing the disease. In patients with multiple medical problems, each problem and its therapy should be distinct. Too often the medical mandate is combined: "stop drinking, stop smoking, and take your pills". The result is noncompliance to them all.

THE PRACTICE OF CHEMOTHERAPY

The revised classification of tuberculosis simplifies the categorization of patients with mycobacterial exposure, infection, and disease and enables the physician to prescribe an effective and safe course of chemotherapy.[5] (See Table I, appendix 1.) Adequate chemotherapeutic regimens produce uniformly excellent results. Prognosis is not determined by factors other than chemotherapy; for example, rest, the amount of fresh air or sunshine, diet, smoking habits, length of hospitalization, and alcohol use or abuse, by themselves, do not influence outcome. All that matters is that the patient receives the medication.

Hospitalization is not required if the patient with newly diagnosed tuberculosis is not toxic and does not require hospitalization for associated medical problems such as trauma and decompensated liver disease.[6] In actual practice, many patients have the diagnosis of pulmonary tuberculosis established during the course of hospitalization. Since the greatest degree of infectivity exists prior to the initiation of the drug therapy, the patient can be safely discharged home after he has demonstrated symptomatic improvement such as a decrease in cough frequency and weight gain, decreased number of organisms in the sputum smear, and no evidence of untoward toxic side effects of his chemotherapy. No improvement usually occurs in the chest x-ray film in the one to two weeks of hospitalization. Prior to discharge, household contacts need to have been investigated and appropriate preventive therapy initiated, if indicated.

CATEGORIZATION AND TREATMENT

A) CATEGORY 0: <u>No tuberculosis exposure, not infected.</u> No therapy necessary.

B) CATEGORY I: <u>Tuberculosis exposure, no evidence of infection.</u> Some contacts not yet proved to be infected (PPD Negative) are candidates for "primary prophylaxis" because the tuberculin skin test may be in the process of conversion.

All household contacts should be considered for such treatment. Primary prophylaxis is standard for children, being especially important for those less than five years of age and essential for neonates. Isoniazid is the only drug with demonstrated effectiveness. The usual duration of treatment is until approximately three months after the contact has been broken, unless the patient changes to Category II.

C) CATEGORY II: Tuberculous infection without disease. The treatment of persons who are infected but do not have disease (PPD Positive; chest roentgenogram and bacteriology negative) is based on the concept that the lifetime risk of developing tuberculosis for an untreated infected person exceeds the risk of taking isoniazid for one year. Positive reactors who are less than 35 years of age are candidates for therapy. Persons older than 35 who have an additional risk factor such as corticosteroid therapy, immunosuppressive therapy or a disease state that impairs the immune response should also be treated.

D) CATEGORY III: Tuberculous infection with disease. Patients who have had tuberculosis and are bacteriologically negative, who have not previously received adequate chemotherapy, should receive isoniazid for one year. Patients who are tuberculin skin test reactors with roentgenographic findings consistent with tuberculous scarring, who have negative bacteriologic studies, should receive isoniazid preventive therapy for one year.

Isoniazid, ethambutol, rifampin, and streptomycin are considered to be first-line or primary drugs for patients with current active tuberculosis (Bacteriology Positive). The most frequently used regimen is isoniazid and ethambutol, for eighteen months, but this is controversial. When the bacterial population is thought to be particularly large (extensive cavitary lesions) or if the patient is from an area where drug-resistant tuberculosis is prevalent, daily streptomycin may be included in the regimen, usually not longer than one to two months, until the bacterial population is reduced.

Rifampin combined with isoniazid is as effective as any three-drug regimen in the treatment of extensive cavitary disease. After the sputum bacteriology becomes negative, ethambutol may be substituted for the rifampin with the total duration of therapy lasting eighteen to twenty-four months.

Patient acceptance, drug toxicity, and cost need to be as important considerations in selecting therapy, as is the efficacy of the drug. An orally administered regimen (isoniazid-rifampin; isoniazid-ethambutol) lends itself to an outpatient program much more than one with streptomycin, which is delivered by painful injections administered by a medical professional. Total cost is the sum of expenditures to the patient by loss of time from work and transportation, as well as program personnel and drug expenses. The actual duration of therapy necessary is under study, but a course of two drugs for eighteen to twenty-four months is almost always successful. At the present time, shorter courses of therapy with isoniazid and rifampin (i. e. 6 to 12 months) are investigational.

Isoniazid and ethambutol are the preferred combination when treatment during pregnancy is necessary.

DISCHARGE OF PATIENTS FROM MEDICAL SURVEILLANCE

The most critical determinant of the course that will be followed by the patient with tuberculosis is the adequacy of the chemotherapy. Experience with drug therapy convincingly indicates that if adequate antituberculous chemotherapy is received by the patient, tubercle bacilli are rapidly eradicated from the sputum and after completion of chemotherapy, relapse is uncommon. Therefore, the long-term surveillance policies designed and utilized in the pre-chemotherapy era are no longer appropriate for tuberculosis patients who have completed adequate drug therapy. Indeed, several reviews of the productivity of long-term follow-up indicate that the majority of relapses are not detected by routine surveillance procedures.

Before discharge from the tuberculosis treatment program, the patient should be instructed as to what symptoms might be associated with reactivity of the tuberculous process and of the importance of the prompt evaluation of these symptoms. The patient should be referred for continuing general health care, making sure that a history of successfully treated pulmonary tuberculosis is noted on his medical record.

TREATMENT OF CHILDREN

The principles of the management of a child with tuberculosis are similar to those which guide the treatment of adults. There are, however, a number of matters unique to children infected with tuberculosis that warrant special consideration. An orderly scheme in diagnosing childhood tuberculosis consists of four procedures: tuberculin skin testing, epidemiologic study of the child's environment, chest x-ray, and attempts to isolate the tubercle bacillus. All exposed children do not contract tuberculosis; in one study the average was 35 percent skin test positivity in households where there was an infectious adult.[8] Rational and successful treatment can be prescribed for both the child and his adult household contacts only after obtaining the appropriate clinical data, skin tests, chest roentgenograms and bacteriology, if indicated, on every member of the household.

The classic x-ray film of a small patch of pneumonitis with enlarged hilar lymph nodes is rarely observed in primary tuberculosis in children; much more common is hilar adenopathy alone. Lobar or segmental disease occurs in primary tuberculosis when enlarging hilar nodes distort the bronchi sufficiently to produce bronchial obstruction and subsequent atelectasis. The atelectatic segment may be only partially collapsed and is easily confused with a pneumonia. Such endobronchial disease with collapse does not represent involvement of a whole segment of lung by tubercle bacilli but rather mechanical obstruction with atelectasis and possibly secondary bacterial invasion. Occasionally, erosion and perforation of a bronchus by an enlarged lymph node allows caseous material to drain into the bronchial system and results in a diffuse tuberculous pneumonia. Miliary disease involves all areas of the lung, is distributed symmetrically, and the lesions characteristically are all of the same size. Cavitation is rare in childhood tuberculosis.

The treatment of children with tuberculosis is based on the same principles as for adults. Two or more drugs should be used when the child is infected with large numbers of bacilli. Para-aminosalicylic acid (PAS) is given to children more often than to adults for the following reasons: children tolerate PAS much better than adults who almost invariably have some degree of gastrointestinal distress after ingesting PAS; rifampin is not approved for use in children although it has been given to children without causing more toxicity than observed in adults; and ethambutol cannot be used in children who are too young to detect visual disturbances.

In children with sensitive organisms, the initial phase of treatment usually consists of isoniazid, PAS and streptomycin (See Table II, Appendix 2, for dosage). After a culture negative state is reached, the streptomycin can be stopped and the isoniazid and PAS continued for twelve months, the isoniazid is then continued alone for an additional six months, making the total treatment period eighteen months.

Children with endobronchial tuberculosis often present some especially challenging questions in the course of their management. The first is whether or not to bronchoscope the child. In recent years, it has been our practice to bronchoscope relatively few children with endobronchial tuberculosis because the diagnosis can usually be established without the procedure which rarely adds anything to the evaluation of such a child. The second question is whether to give concomitant corticosteroids to such children. Almost all children with endobronchial tuberculosis follow a benign course while receiving antituberculous chemotherapy and corticosteroids should be reserved for those very few patients who demonstrate progressive and massive collapse with resulting symptoms and signs of pulmonary insufficiency. The final problem in managing the child with endobronchial tuberculosis is found in the subsequent chest roentgenograms after treatment has been instituted. Although the patient may be asymptomatic, afebrile and gaining weight, the two to three month follow-up chest x-ray films may demonstrate either lack of improvement or even, on occasion, slight worsening of the atelectasis. Such a finding need not represent unfavorable progress and is not an indication for corticosteroid therapy unless it is associated with other clinical evidence of deterioration such as weight loss, fever and hypoxemia.

A lumbar puncture probably should be done on every child admitted to the hospital with bacteriologically positive disease. Central nervous system tuberculosis can be present in children with few or no systemic symptoms or signs such as headache or nuchal rigidity.

COMPLICATIONS OF TUBERCULOSIS

RESPIRATORY FAILURE

Arterial blood gas values have been thought to be near normal in patients with pulmonary tuberculosis because of concomitant impairment of ventilation and perfusion and the maintenance of normal ventilation to perfusion relationships. In some patients, however, this is not true and life-threatening hypoxemia, with or without CO_2 retention, has been observed in a number of patients with bacteriologically positive pulmonary tuberculosis.[9] There is considerable mortality associated with the respiratory failure found in patients with pulmonary tuberculosis but with prompt oxygen therapy, and rarely a period of mechanical ventilatory support, there are long-term survivors.

The principles of management are the same as for other patients with respiratory failure. Arterial blood gas analyses should be performed on tuberculosis patients with extensive pulmonary disease so that abnormalities of gas exchange will not be missed.

FEVER AND NON-TUBERCULOUS SEPTICEMIA

The fever that is so common a symptom and sign in patients with bacteriologically positive pulmonary tuberculosis is thought to be due to the absorption of tuberculoprotein by the hypersensitive host and to the products of disintegrating leukocytes. After appropriate antituberculous chemotherapy is initiated, the patient's fever usually decreases at the rate of approximately one degree Fahrenheit per week. For example, if the patient's afternoon temperature elevations reached 102°-F the first few days after diagnosis and institution of chemotherapy, one would expect the elevations to be 101° in one week, 100° in two weeks. However, there may be considerable variations, both slower and more rapid defervescence, from this general rule.

Since fever is so common in patients with pulmonary tuberculosis, non-tuberculous infections may be overlooked. This is a real problem, and non-tuberculous septicemia has been discovered in a number of patients with active tuberculous infection. The organisms identified as the cause of such septicemias include *Pneumococci*, *Klebsiella* and *Serratia*.[10] The most common sources of the septicemia have been the lungs and genitourinary tract. With appropriate antibiotics these patients improved rapidly. Therefore, all toxic, febrile patients with bacteriologically positive pulmonary tuberculosis should have sputum, urine and blood cultures obtained so as to avoid missing a potentially curable non-tuberculous septicemia.

HEMOPTYSIS

Hemoptysis may be infrequent and insignificant or massive and fatal in patients with pulmonary tuberculosis. The erosion of an artery in a thick-walled cavity, Rasmussen's aneurysm, is associated with severe hemoptysis because these vessels are derived from bronchial arteries and reflect systemic arterial pressures. An aspergilloma in a tuberculous cavity may also cause hemoptysis. Patients with hemoptysis due to either a Rasmussen's aneurysm or an aspergilloma are usually bacteriologically negative with respect to *M. tuberculosis*. However, massive hemoptysis may occur in patients with bacteriologically positive pulmonary tuberculosis whose chest roentgenograms demonstrate fibernodular infiltration without cavitation.[11]

The management of patients with pulmonary tuberculosis and massive hemoptysis is difficult and controversial. Some favor a conservative approach with rest and supportive measures such as blood transfusions and rarely perform emergency surgery. Others have advocated a more aggressive approach with early surgical intervention. Our approach is to hospitalize pulmonary tuberculosis patients with major hemoptysis and perform fiberoptic bronchoscopy in an attempt to locate the source of the bleeding. It should be noted, however, that the bleeding can be of such severity that all of the airways are filled with blood and the precise source of bleeding frequently cannot be identified. Following bronchoscopy the patient is placed at bedrest and hopefully the bleeding stops. The ideal candidate for surgery is one who stops bleeding and who has an isolated fibrotic lobe as the source of the bleeding and otherwise normal appearing and functioning lung parenchyma. Such an individual could have a lobectomy at a time when he is not bleeding. However, such patients are the exception. Many patients have diffuse disease with markedly impaired pulmonary function. Newer techniques such as bronchial artery embolization may offer hope for patients who suffer from an episode of massive hemoptysis.[12]

EXTRAPULMONARY TUBERCULOSIS

Tuberculosis infection has been found in virtually every organ of the body. The ingestion route of infection, common in the days of unpasteurized milk, is rarely a problem in countries in which pasteurization is routine. The pathogenesis of extrapulmonary tuberculosis usually is as follows: after the introduction of the infectious droplet nuclei into the lungs and widespread hematogenous dissemination, a latent period that may last from brief periods to many years occurs before the infection becomes bacteriologically active in kidney, bone, meninges, peritoneum or pericardium.

The principles of antituberculous chemotherapy used to treat pulmonary infection with tuberculosis also apply to extrapulmonary tuberculosis. Two effective drugs for eighteen to twenty-four months is almost always successful in treating drug sensitive extrapulmonary organisms. Special aspects of the therapy of extrapulmonary tuberculosis include corticosteroids and surgery. Concomitant chemotherapy has made surgical procedures such as drainage and removal of caseous material and stabilization of diseased bones not only safe, but in most instances, unnecessary.

GENITOURINARY TUBERCULOSIS

Pyuria, hematuria and proteinuria may be found as manifestations of renal tuberculosis. However, most patients with renal tuberculosis have no symptoms and few or no urinary abnormalities other than a urine culture positive for Mycobacterium tuberculosis. Tuberculous salpingitis is the most common type of genital tuberculosis in the female, while in the male the prostate is most frequently involved; the seminal vesicles and epididymis are less frequently infected. Sinus formation, calcification and obstruction may complicate genitourinary tuberculosis. Chemotherapy for eighteen to twenty-four months is almost always successful and surgery may be required.

SKELETAL TUBERCULOSIS

Tuberculosis of the spine may cause destruction sufficient to lead to collapse of the involved vertebra with resulting deformity such as a gibbus and may even produce paraplegia. Involvement of the spine may be associated with a paraspinal abscess. Chemotherapy has limited and often eliminated the necessity for immobilization and surgical procedures such as abscess drainage and spinal fusion, even in patients with neurological impairment.[13]

CENTRAL NERVOUS SYSTEM TUBERCULOSIS

The symptoms and signs of central nervous system tuberculosis are related to toxemia, meningeal irritation, increased intracranial pressure, compression or direct involvement of nervous tissue, hydrocephalus and infarction.[14] Fever and headache are prominent early symptoms. The hyponatremia of the inappropriate antidiuretic hormone syndrome is often associated with CNS tuberculosis and may cause abnormalities in mental status. Meningeal signs and changes in personality or sensorium such as apathy, irritability, and lethargy then appear. Vomiting and strabismus may be fairly early findings. In the later stages, confusion progresses to coma, and cranial nerve palsies, paraplegia and hemiplegia are found. In infants, a tense fontanelle without meningeal signs is more usual; and in children, the only meningeal sign may be nuchal rigidity. On funduscopic examination, papilledema may be observed, and rarely, choroidal tubercles may be seen. Although these symptoms typically develop and worsen over a period of several days, development may be acute or occur over a period of a number of weeks.

The cerebrospinal fluid is usually clear and colorless, but occasionally may be xanthochromic or slightly cloudy. On standing for a few hours, a pellicle, like a fine wisp of cotton, may appear in the fluid. One has the best chance of observing acid-fast bacilli on direct smear in the pellicle although they are infrequently found. The cerebrospinal fluid pressure is uniformly increased except under special circumstances where spinal block (in which the thickened meninges of the spinal cord prevent the circulation of cerebrospinal fluid) occurs; then it may be normal or even low. The cells are increased in number from slightly so to several hundred or a thousand and usually are predominantly mononuclear; a majority of polymorphonuclears are occasionally seen in the early stages. Typically, the count is 50-500 WBC/mm^3. The protein is elevated varying from minimally so to a gram or more (typically 50-400 mg%). The sugar is usually mildly to moderately reduced.

Evidence of concomitant miliary tuberculosis (usually by chest film) is almost diagnostic and evidence of an active tuberculous focus elsewhere.

MILIARY TUBERCULOSIS

Miliary tuberculosis is an illness produced by an acute dissemination of tubercle bacilli via the blood stream. In the lung this process is manifested by the appearance of tiny, discrete foci rather uniformly distributed. The shadows seen on the chest x-ray film may be so small that they are barely visible, or not seen at all. It is not certain whether the size of the miliary lesions is related to the number of tubercle bacilli discharged in the blood stream or to the amount of toxic material derived from the bacilli.

In children the diagnosis of miliary tuberculosis is relatively simple; but, in the middle-aged and elderly, who frequently have concomitant major illnesses, the disease often develops insidiously and may present few characteristic symptoms or signs. Miliary tuberculosis may be missed during the gross autopsy examination and a histologic examination may be necessary for the diagnosis, even at autopsy. Skin testing, chest roentgenograms and specimens from extrapulmonary sites are all helpful in establishing the diagnosis. A transbronchial biopsy, performed during fiberoptic bronchoscopy, has proven to be highly efficacious in diagnosing miliary tuberculosis and has been an important addition to the methods for diagnosing the disease.[15] Hematologic and hepatic abnormalities often are present and bone marrow and liver biopsy may establish the diagnosis of miliary tuberculosis. Body cavity fluids, when involved with tuberculosis, may demonstrate abnormalities highly suggestive of tuberculosis and pleural and peritoneal biopsy can also be diagnostic.

Chemotherapy for patients with miliary tuberculosis is not different from other patients with bacteriologically positive tuberculous disease.

CORTICOSTEROIDS AS AN ADJUNCT TO TREATMENT

Adrenal insufficiency is the only physiologically valid clinical situation in which corticosteroids are administered to a patient with tuberculosis. We have never seen an instance of adrenal insufficiency in a patient with bacteriologically positive tuberculosis, although, on numerous occasions, the diagnosis has been considered because of symptoms and signs identical to those of adrenal insufficiency such as weakness, dehydration, hypotension, and hyponatremia. Inappropriate ADH syndrome and a variety of electrolyte disturbances have been reported but, despite appropriate biochemical determinations, adrenal insufficiency has not been documented. This does not mean that dehydrated, hypotensive tuberculosis patients should not be investigated for adrenal insufficiency; we will continue to do so. It just means that we have not yet observed it.

Recommendations advocating the use of corticosteroids in tuberculosis have included tuberculous pericarditis and meningitis, endobronchial tuberculosis in children and the toxic, hypoxemic patient with extensive pulmonary tuberculosis. Improvement following cortocosteroid therapy has been documented in a small controlled study on patients with tuberculous pericarditis.[16]

In tuberculous meningitis, survival has not been improved by the addition of corticosteroids to adequate antituberculous chemotherapy although there may be a decrease in the cerebrospinal fluid pressure and subjective improvement associated with corticosteroid therapy.

The outcome of endobronchial tuberculosis in children is sufficiently favorable following the institution of chemotherapy, and corticosteroid therapy is not usually necessary in such patients.

Although all the data are anecdotal, we agree with those who administer corticosteroids (i. e. prednisone, 40 to 60 mg.

per day) to the debilitated, toxic, hypotensive, hypoxemic adult with extensive pulmonary tuberculosis. Prednisone may benefit such a patient by suppressing toxicity and prolonging life for a period of time sufficient for the antituberculous chemotherapy to improve pulmonary gas exchange and for the patient to regain strength. Our policy is to give corticosteroids to such a patient in the hopes of obtaining this "extra" time; yet we do it with the knowledge that there is no controlled study that supports this theory.

SUPERVISED INTERMITTENT THERAPY

Standard regimens of daily antituberculous chemotherapy are successful in almost every patient with drug sensitive organisms who completes eighteen to twenty-four months of therapy. However, failure to adhere to these long-term courses of medication is the most important cause of treatment failure. Frequently, adequate treatment can only be assured in such patients by directly observing the swallowing of the pills and the injection of parenteral medicines.

Intermittent chemotherapy should be used only after a successful initial phase of daily treatment which usually takes two to four months and is reached after one or more negative sputum cultures have been obtained. When intermittent supervised therapy is used, twice weekly therapy is recommended because twice weekly is superior to once weekly and not significantly less effective than three times a week.[17] Safe and effective twice weekly regimens have consisted of isoniazid-ethambutol and isoniazid-streptomycin. Intermittent rifampin therapy has been associated with considerable toxicity. The dosages for twice weekly supervised intermittent therapy are:

Isoniazid	15 mg per kg - oral
and	
Ethambutol	50 mg per kg - oral

or

Isoniazid	15 mg per kg - oral
and	
Streptomycin	25 & 30 mg per kg - intramuscular

Intermittent therapy is almost totally effective if continued for eighteen months after the first negative culture is obtained. The missed treatment rate should be kept lower than

5 percent, although successful courses of therapy have been reported when the missed treatment rate has been as high as 10 percent. It is important to realize that intermittent therapy is not presently considered to be standard therapy and is reserved for unusually difficult treatment problems. We wish to stress that initial daily therapy, until one or more negative sputum cultures are obtained, is mandatory in a supervised intermittent therapy program.

The emergence of a drug-resistant organism has not been found with any more frequency after intermittent, rather than daily, therapy. No adverse reactions have been reported to intermittent ethambutol. Rare occurrences of peripheral neuritis have been noted, presumably secondary to isoniazid, and pyridoxine hydrochloride should be routinely given. Vertigo, giddiness and ataxia have necessitated the discontinuation of intermittent streptomycin injections in up to 10 percent of patients.

ILLUSTRATIVE CASES

CASE 1: PRIMARY TREATMENT

This 25-year-old male construction worker was referred in February, 1976, because of a productive cough and weight loss. He denied hemoptysis and chest pain but stated that his cough had become progressively more severe for the past four months and that for the preceding two months he had experienced night sweats. He denied any recent known exposure to tuberculosis but believed that a relative had had tuberculosis and also that he had been told that his skin test was positive when he was a teenager. He had not received prior treatment with isoniazid. He lived with his wife and three-month-old son. He used alcohol socially.

Physical examination revealed a pleasant young man who was not toxic and appeared to be in no distress. The only abnormal physical findings were rhonchi and rales over the left hemithorax and a temperature of 101°F. His chest x-ray is shown in Figure 4.1.

A PPD (5 TU) skin test produced 15 mm of induration. The sputum smear was markedly positive for acid-fast bacilli. Sputum was sent for culture for M. tuberculosis and blood chemistries were drawn (Table 4.1).

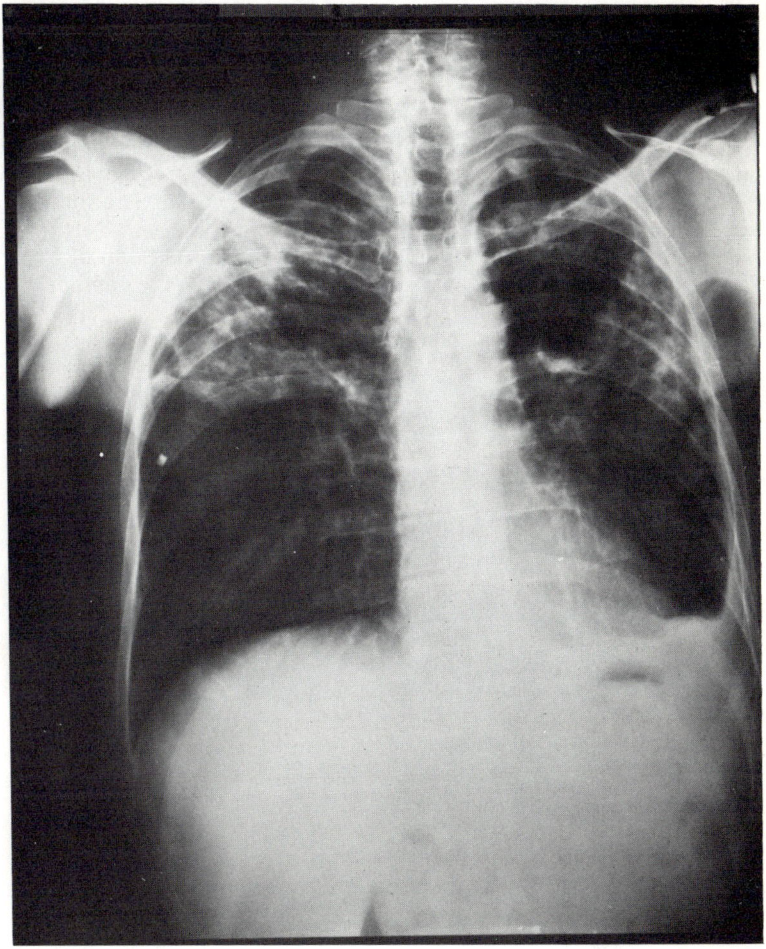

FIG. 4. 1: The chest roentgenogram of 25-year-old male (Case 1) at the time of initial diagnosis of pulmonary tuberculosis.

TABLE 4.1

Date	Weight	Sputum Smear	Culture Results	SGOT	SGPT	Total Bilirubin	Alkaline Phosphatase
2/25/76	164 lbs.	3+	4+	15	24	0.3	75
3/10/76		1+	3+	155	30	0.5	80
3/25/76		1+	10 colonies	59	16	0.7	84
4/7/76		Neg.	1 colony	96	39	0.9	72
5/5/76	180 lbs.	Neg.	Neg.	65	23	1.3	141
6/2/76		Neg.	Neg.	131	40	0.9	106
7/14/76		Neg.	Neg.	31	68	1.1	80
8/12/76		Neg.	Neg.	75	21	0.8	77
9/10/76	185 lbs.	Neg.	Neg.	63	45	0.5	75

We elected to treat the patient entirely as an outpatient with daily isoniazid and rifampin, and he was instructed to return the next day with his wife and child. Another sputum was obtained for culture when he returned the next day. Both his wife and child were well and both had a negative PPD skin test. The mother and child were placed on isoniazid preventive therapy. Three months later their PPD skin tests were still negative and the patient was then smear negative, so isoniazid therapy was discontinued for the wife and child. The patient's fellow construction workers were not skin tested.

The patient did very well. He was a member of a research protocol and for this reason liver function tests were obtained monthly (See Table 4. 1). The isoniazid and rifampin were continued for six months after which ethambutol was substituted for the rifampin. He received the drug therapy for a total of twenty-four months and was then discharged with a copy of his record and his chest roentgenogram (Figure 4. 2) and instructions to return if he noticed any symptoms of reactivation, such as productive cough and weight loss.

Comment: This patient demonstrates the marked reduction in the disruption to the life of a patient treated as an outpatient with modern chemotherapy in comparison to previous lengthy sanatorium hospitalizations. He did not have to leave his wife, child or home or lose his job. His wife and child received primary prophylaxis (Category I: Tuberculosis exposure, no evidence of infection) for three months after which their isoniazid was discontinued because their PPD skin tests remained non-reactive and the source case was bacteriologically negative.

The local Health Department was consulted and because the patient's household contacts were PPD negative, it was decided not to skin test his fellow construction workers. The reasoning was that because he had not infected his household contacts whose exposure was far greater and indoors, it was unlikely that he had infected his fellow workers. His exposure to fellow workers was much shorter and outdoors, and the chance of infection in the construction workers was extremely remote.

Finally, Table 4. 1 is a good example of why not to perform routine monitoring liver function tests. The SGOT varied between 15 and 131, the SGPT between 16 and 68, the alkaline phosphatase between 72 to 106 and the bilirubin between 0. 3 to 1. 3. Since he was asymptomatic during this entire period, there was no indication for obtaining these tests, which were required by a research protocol, and needless aggravation of all concerned in his care could have been avoided. Just what the fluctuations

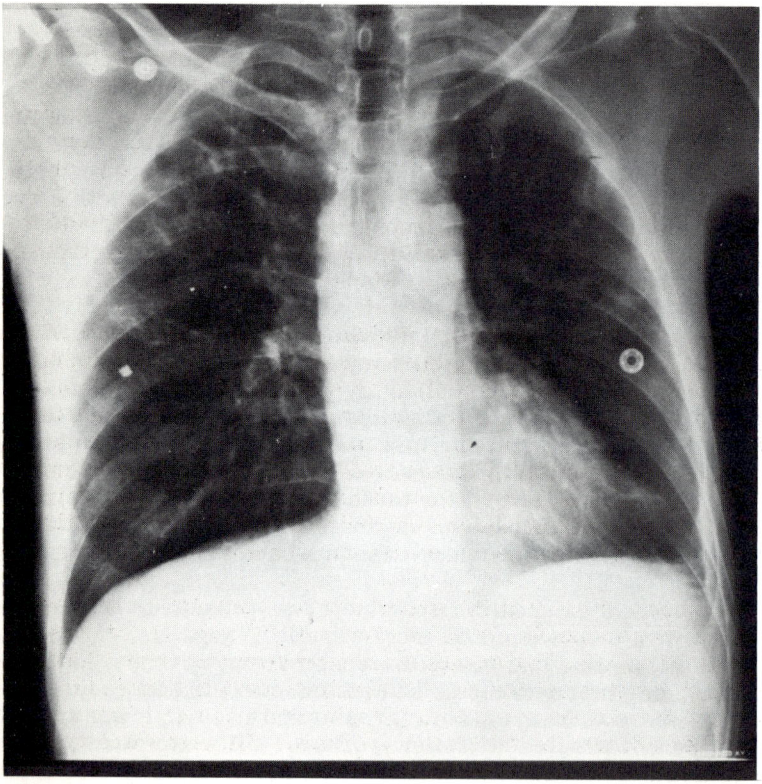

FIG. 4. 2: Chest film in Case 1 at end of chemotherapy program revealing marked clearing of infiltrates.

in his liver function tests represented is not apparent; possibilities include "heavy" social ethanol consumption, laboratory error and drug interference with the test determinations.

CASE 2: PRIMARY TREATMENT

M. M. was twelve months old, when he received a tuberculin skin test because his uncle, who lived in the same household, was hospitalized with bacteriologically positive pulmonary tuberculosis. A PPD intermediate skin test resulted in 25 mm. of induration and a chest x-ray film was abnormal (Figure 4.3). Tomograms (Figure 4.4) reveal right upper lobe collapses. No symptoms could be elicited from the child's mother who was surprised to learn that he was ill. Physical examination was within normal limits; he was in the nineteenth percentile for weight.

The child was hospitalized to initiate therapy which consisted of isoniazid, PAS and streptomycin daily during his two weeks in the hospital. After discharge, INH and PAS were continued and a visiting nurse continued the streptomycin five times a week for two months and directly observed that the child and the other members of the family received their medication.

In the hospital, all laboratory studies were normal except for a normocytic, normochromic anemia. Gastric washings were obtained for culture but no sputum was obtained. The child was bronchoscoped at which time the right upper lobe was almost completely occluded by external compression. The bronchial mucosa was red but bronchial washings were smear and culture negative. The gastric washings also failed to grow out Mycobacterium tuberculosis.

Isoniazid and PAS were continued for one year and isoniazid alone for a total of eighteen months. All therapy was then stopped, at which time all household contacts were either on therapy or were skin test negative. His outpatient visits revealed normal growth and development. Serial chest x-ray films demonstrated slow initial improvement, but later, complete resolution with a normal chest x-ray film (Figures 4.5 and 4.6).

Comment: This child was discovered to have pulmonary tuberculosis during screening of all household contacts of a patient with bacteriologically positive pulmonary tuberculosis. Unlike adults, this child tolerated PAS therapy, as many children do. It should be noted that he was asymptomatic throughout his course of chemotherapy despite rather dramatic chest x-ray

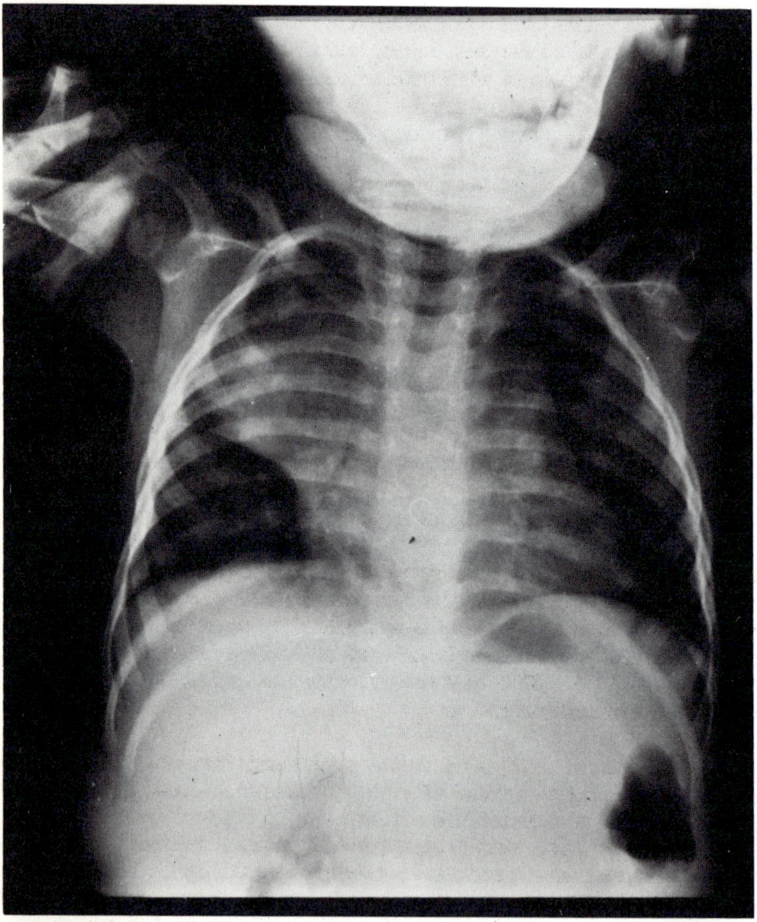

FIG. 4.3: Chest x-ray of Case 2 revealing partial right upper lobe atelectasis.

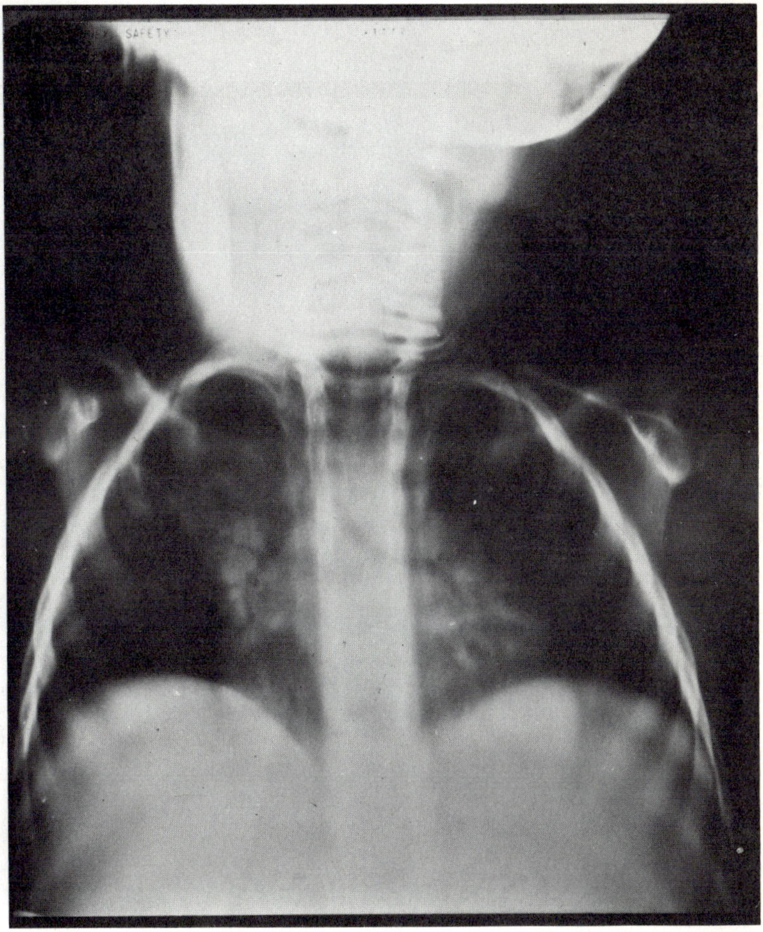

FIG. 4.4: Tomogram of hilum in Case 2 revealing marked right hilar adenopathy and right upper lobe atelectasis secondary to extrinsic bronchial obstruction related to primary M. tuberculosis infection.

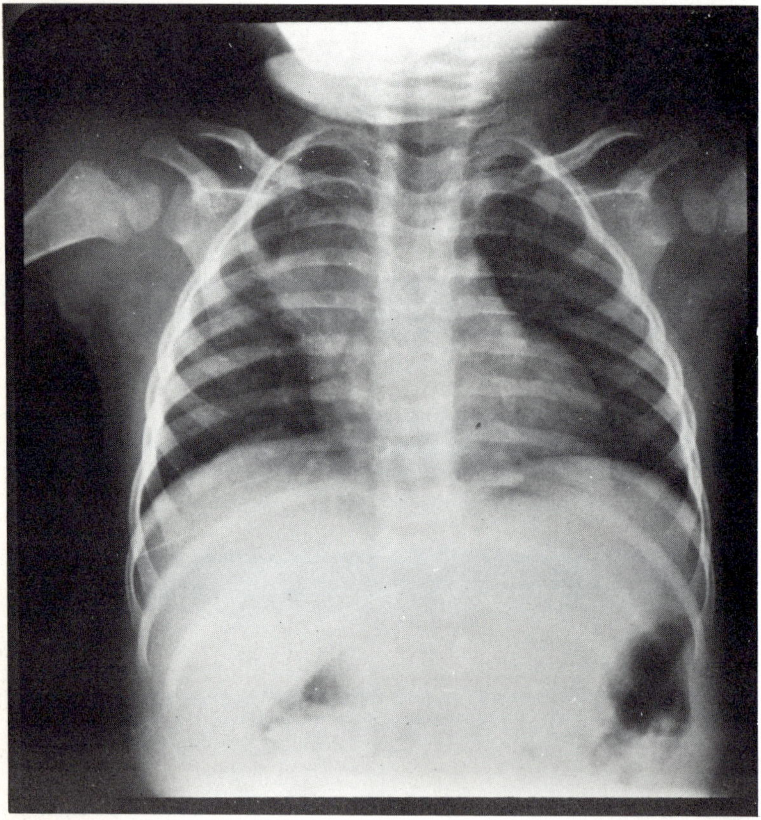

FIG. 4.5: Chest film of Case 2 after three months of antituberculous chemotherapy.

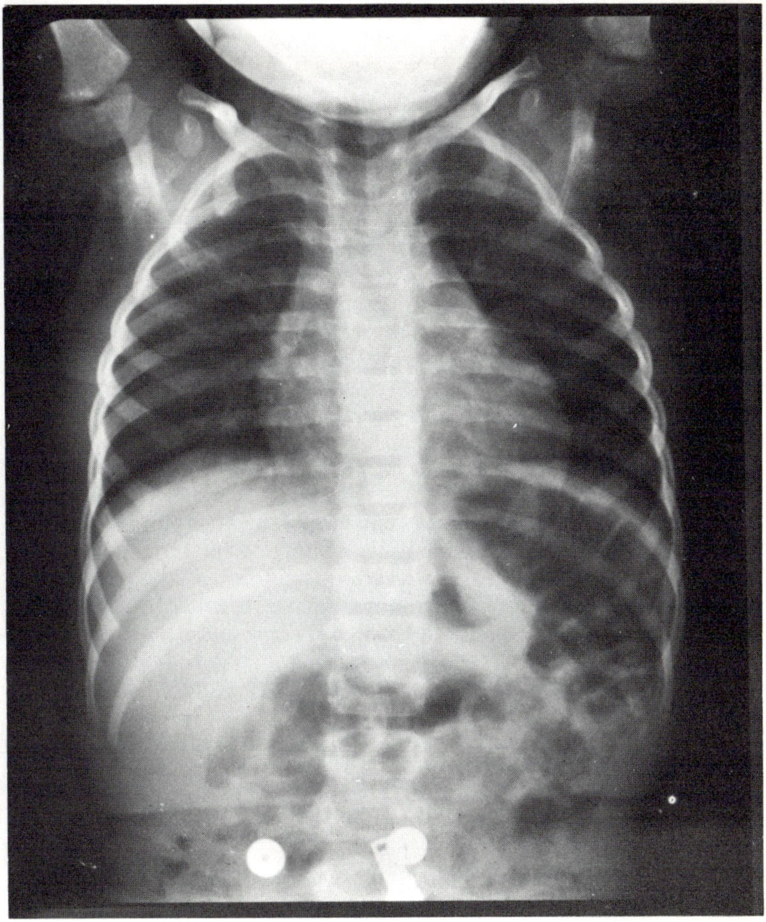

FIG. 4. 6: Chest roentgenogram of Case 2 after four months of antituberculous chemotherapy.

findings which actually progressed while on therapy. All that is needed in such a situation is to ascertain that the patient is receiving his medications, which was done, and not to change his medication. If a pediatric bronchoscopist is available, these children may be bronchoscoped, but such examinations are not essential. Finally, all such children should have a spinal fluid examination to exclude the possibility of concomitant tuberculosis meningitis.

CASE 3: PRIMARY TREATMENT

M.P. was two years old when she was brought to an Emergency Room because she was noted to be limping on her right leg. The mother stated that the child began to limp three months previously and that she noted that she did not straighten her right leg when she walked. She had suffered no known trauma and she did not complain of pain in the hip or knee. She played normally and despite her limp was active at home. Physical examination revealed a slight but definite swelling, that was not red or tender, along the right side of the lower spine. There was moderate kyphosis and the right knee was held flexed with a slight external rotation of the hip. There was full range of motion of the right knee and hip. There was no neurological deficit.

The admission chest x-ray was normal. Spine x-rays (Figure 4.7)reavealed destruction of the body of the fourth and fifth lumbar vertebra. An intravenous pyelogram (Figure 4.8) showed normally functioning kidneys and ureters but the bladder and left ureter were displaced anteriorly by a mass. An inferior venocavagram demonstrated that there was a paravertebral mass displacing the inferior vena cava anteriorly (Figure 4.9).

A PPD skin test resulted in 20 mm induration. A review of the family history revealed that the grandmother had been hospitalized with tuberculosis shortly after the child's birth, apparently had taken her medication irregularly and had recently moved away.

The patient was hospitalized for six weeks while she received isoniazid, PAS and streptomycin. A neurological consultant found no neurological deficit and the child was not placed in traction but allowed to move freely around the ward and the playroom. After discharge the patient received isoniazid and PAS for eighteen months and isoniazid for a total of twenty-four months. The swelling and kyphosis improved gradually over a four-month period and the child no longer limped after six

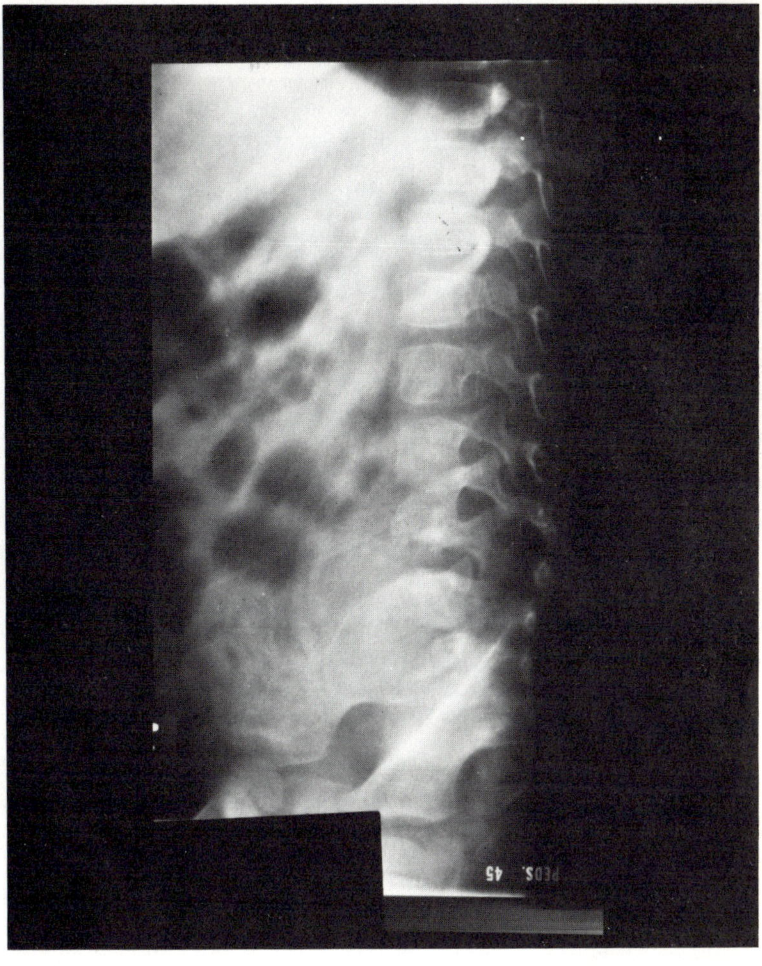

FIG. 4.7: Spine x-rays of Case 3 revealing destruction of the body of the fourth and fifth lumbar vertebrae by tuberculosis.

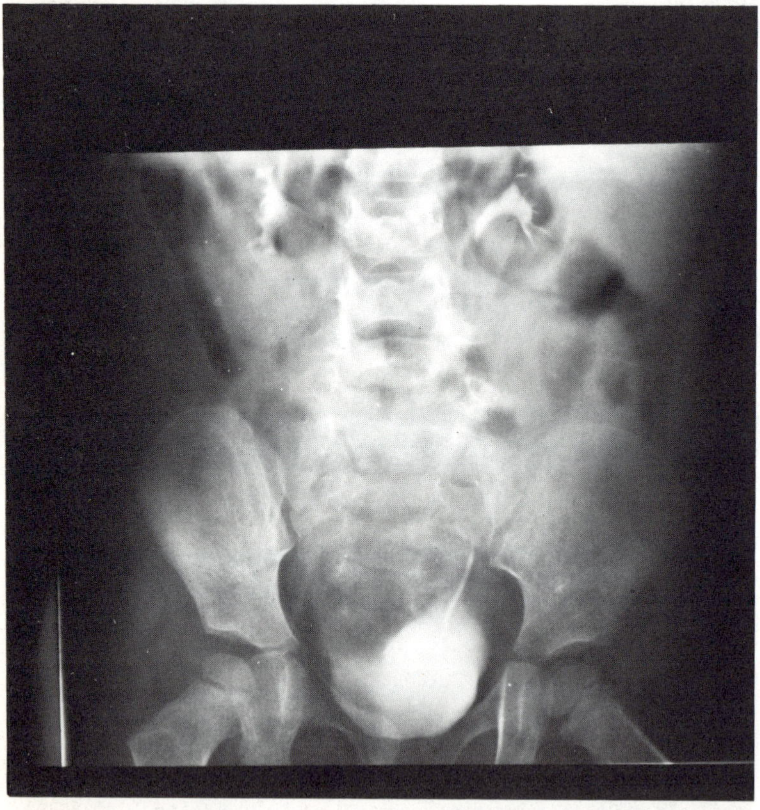

FIG. 4.8: Intravenous pyelogram of Case 3 revealing anterior and leftward displacement of the bladder and left ureter by a paraspinal mass.

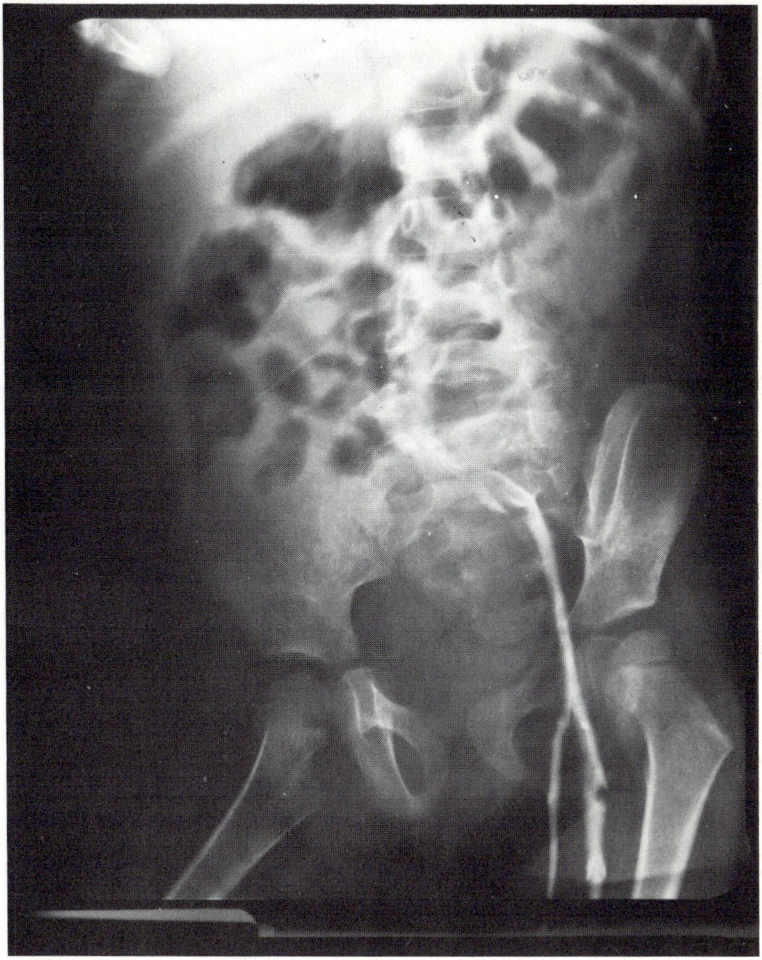

FIG. 4.9: An inferior venacavogram done in Case 3 reveals anterior displacement of the inferior vena cava by the paravertebral mass (cold abscess).

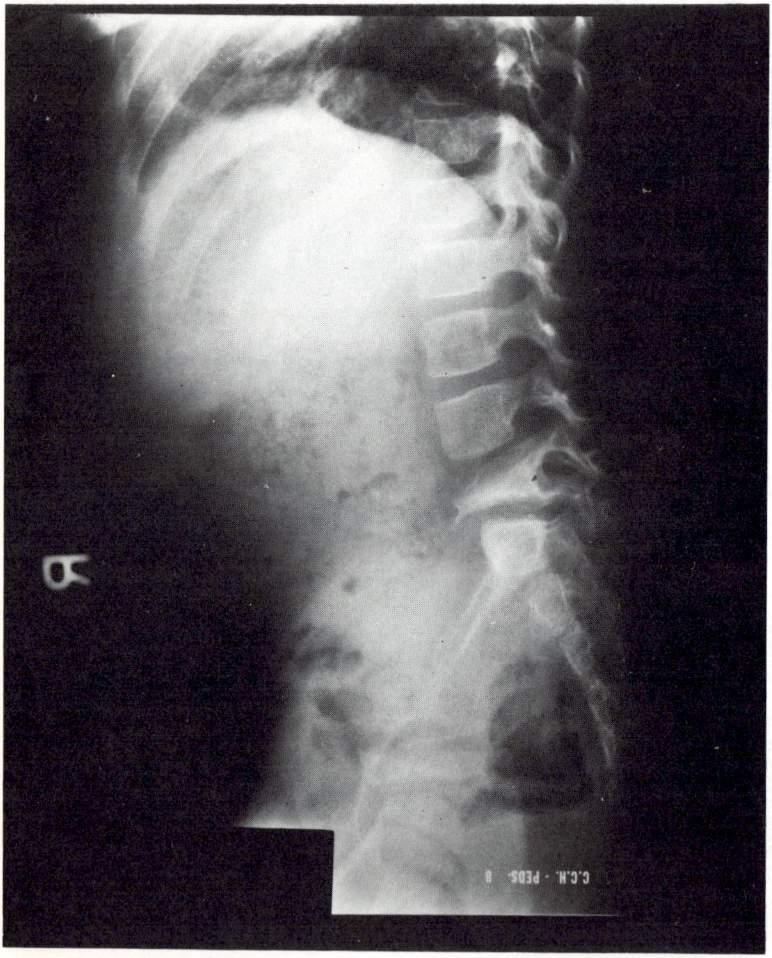

FIG. 4.10: The spine x-ray in Case 3 reveals healing and sclerotic reaction in lumbar spine after twenty-three months of chemotherapy for tuberculosis.

months. Follow-up spine x-ray (Figure 4.10) demonstrated growth and considerable sclerotic reaction.

Comment: This child presented with the symptoms, signs and roentgenographic findings typical of Pott's disease. There was little need for tissue or bacteriologic confirmation of tuberculosis of the spine because of her clinical manifestations as well as her positive PPD and the fact that there was a known bacteriologically positive household contact. Controlled studies of the variety of medical and surgical procedures utilized in the past for Pott's disease have been re-evaluated with large numbers of patients in several underdeveloped countries.[13] Modern chemotherapy makes radical surgery and even abscess drainage and immobilization unnecessary.

CASE 4: SUPERVISED INTERMITTENT TREATMENT

S. S. was 41 years old when he first diagnosed as having pulmonary tuberculosis in 1970. He was admitted to a tuberculosis sanatorium where therapy was initiated with isoniazid, PAS and streptomycin. After six months he left the sanatorium against medical advice. From 1970 to 1976 he was hospitalized on at least nine occasions. His sputum was smear and culture positive on every admission, as it was at the time of his infrequent outpatient clinic visits. Sensitivity studies consistently demonstrated that his organisms were susceptible to all the drugs tested. Beginning in February, 1976, he was hospitalized for two months and daily treatment with isoniazid, rifampin and streptomycin produced negative sputum smears for mycobacteria after ten weeks. His admission chest roentgenogram is shown in Figure 4.11.

He was then started on a supervised intermittent regimen of isoniazid and ethambutol. Although he was drunk at almost every visit and usually required transportation assistance to and from the outpatient clinic, he missed only a few appointments. He has continued sputum negative, gained 35 pounds and demonstrated a marked improvement in his chest roentgenogram (Figure 4.12).

Comment: Supervised intermittent chemotherapy following an initial course of daily drug therapy cured this patient of pulmonary tuberculosis after he had been a treatment failure and had remained sputum positive for more than six years.

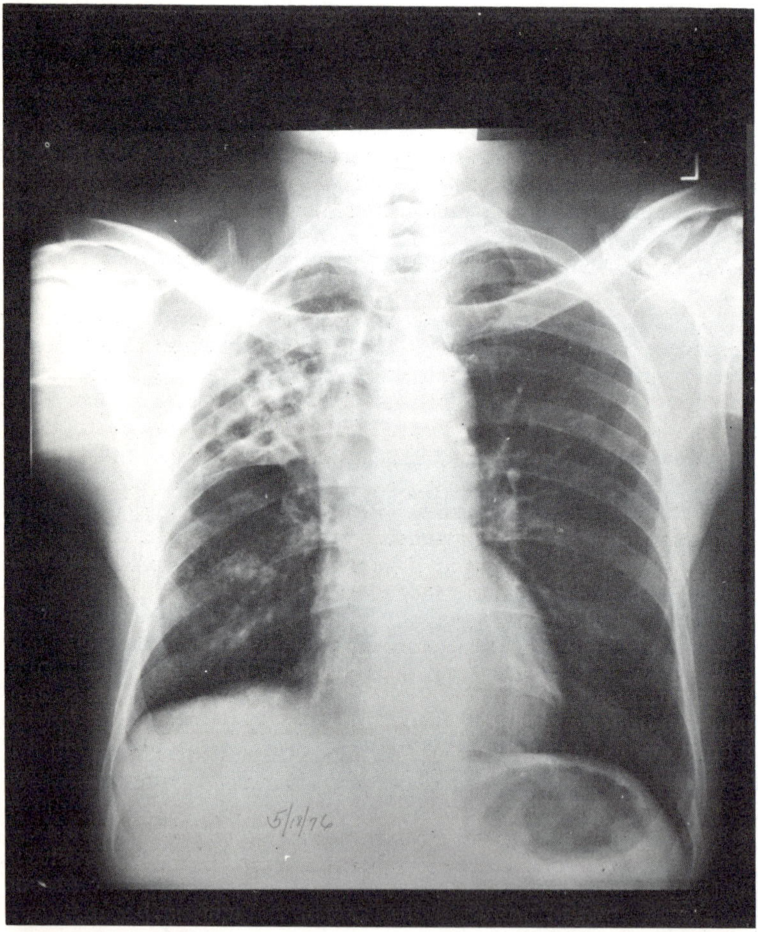

FIG. 4.11: The chest roentgenogram of the patient described in Case 4 reveals tuberculosis of the right lung with cavitation and loss of volume in the right upper lobe.

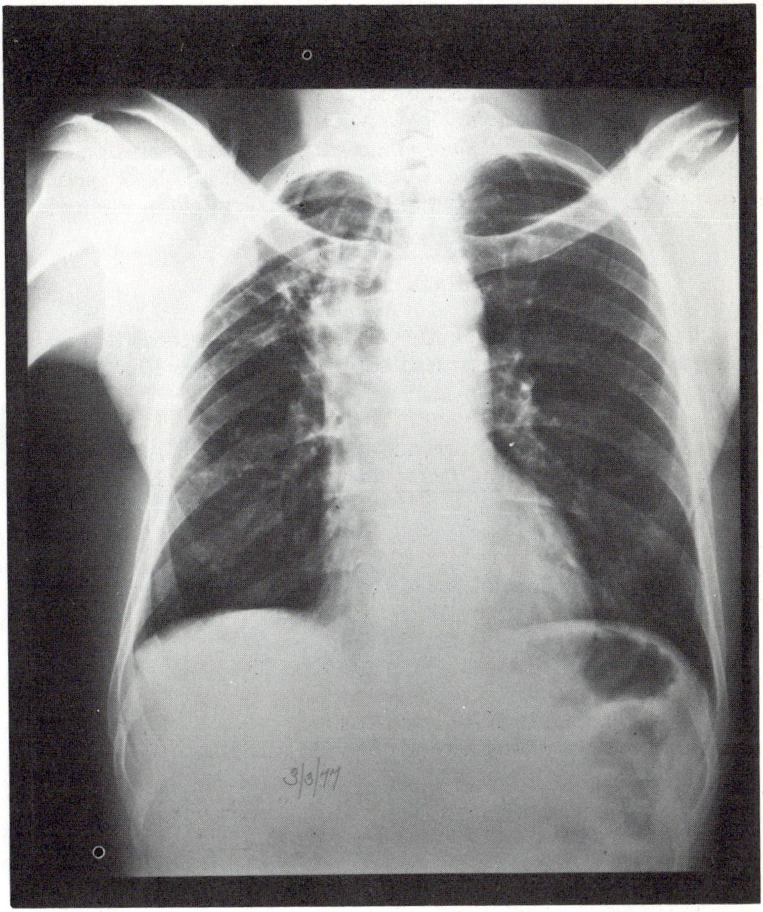

FIG. 4.12: After 10 months of antituberculous chemotherapy, there is marked improvement in the appearance of the right lung on x-ray.

Those caring for patients with tuberculosis must recognize not only the obvious consequences to the personal health of such individuals, but also the real potential for such a patient to infect others. Until programs such as supervised intermittent chemotherapy are available for all patients who fail conventional, daily, unsupervised therapy, any hopes of eradicating tuberculosis are unrealistic.

It should be noted from this patient's history that the reason for success was the provision of transportation and the supervision of his therapy. It was clearly not sophisticated medical decisions, but rather, doggedly persistent efforts by staff to locate this severe and self-destructive alcoholic and to supervise his chemotherapy that led to the arrest of his disease.

REFERENCES

1. Johnston RF, Wildrick KH: The impact of chemotherapy on the care of patients with tuberculosis. Am Rev Respir Dis 109:636, 1974.

2. Cannetti G: Host factors and chemotherapy of tuberculosis. IN: Chemotherapy of Tuberculosis. London, Butterworths, 1964, p. 175.

3. Mitchell JR, Zimmerman HJ, Ishak KG, et al.: Isoniazid, liver injury: Clinical spectrum, pathology, and probable pathogenesis. Ann Int Med 84:181, 1976.

4. Sanders WE: Rifampin, Ann Int Med 85:82, 1976.

5. Bailey WC, Raleigh JW, and Turner JAP: Treatment of mycobacterial disease. Am Rev Respir Dis 115:185, 1977.

6. Sbarbaro JA: Tuberculosis: The new challenge to the practicing clinician. Chest 68:436, 1975.

7. Reichman LB: Routine follow-up of inactive tuberculosis: A practice that has been abandoned. Am Rev Respir Dis 108:1442, 1973.

8. Loudon RG and Spohn SK: Cough frequency and infectivity in patients with pulmonary tuberculosis. Am Rev Respir Dis 99:109, 1969.

9. Agarwal MK, Muthuswamy PP, Banner AS, et al.: Res-

piratory failure in pulmonary tuberculosis. Chest 72:605, 1977.

10. Agarwal MK, Muthuswamy PP, Banner AS, et al.: Septicemia: Occurrence with bacteriologically positive pulmonary tuberculosis. JAMA 238:2297, 1977.

11. Middleton JR, Sen P, Lange M, et al.: Death-producing hemoptysis in tuberculosis. Chest 72:601, 1977.

12. Bookstein JJ, Moser KM, Kalafer ME, et al.: The role of bronchial arteriography and therapeutic embolization in hemoptysis. Chest 72:658, 1977.

13. Tuli SM: Results of treatment of spinal tuberculosis by "Middle-Path" regime. J Bone Joint Surg 57:13, 1975.

14. Kocen RS and Parsons M: Neurological complications of tuberculosis. Quart J Med 39:17, 1970.

15. Sahn SA and Neff TA: Miliary tuberculosis. Am J Med 56:495, 1974.

16. Rooney JJ, Grocco JA, and Lyons HA: Tuberculous pericarditis. Ann Int Med 72:73, 1970.

17. Sbarbaro JA, Barlow PB, Craig MW, et al.: Intermittent chemotherapy for adults with tuberculosis. Am Rev Respir Dis 110:374, 1974.

CHAPTER V:

RESISTANT TUBERCULOSIS

The demonstration by in vitro susceptibility tests that a patient's tubercule bacilli survive and multiply in the presence of elevated concentrations of antituberculosis drugs, indicates resistance. There are two types of drug resistance. The first is Primary Drug Resistance which is defined as the demonstration of lack of susceptibility of a patient's tubercle bacilli to a drug that the patient previously has not received. Such primary drug resistance is attributed to the transmission of a drug-resistant organism and not as a consequence of previous antituberculosis therapy. It is most commonly observed in patients coming from areas of inadequate chemotherapy; for example, Korea, Vietnam, parts of Latin America and some ghetto areas in the United States. The overall incidence of primary drug resistance has remained unchanged in the United States for the last few years. However, as Lester and others caution, primary drug resistance must be considered possible in any area or group in which antituberculosis chemotherapy has consisted of inappropriate regimens or where lack of patient compliance to therapy is recognized.[1]

The second type of drug resistance is termed Acquired or Secondary Drug Resistance. This is due to previous treatment with a drug that was either inadequately prescribed or, if the instructions were appropriate, the drug was irregularly received by the patient. There is agreement that, once resistance to a specific antituberculosis drug has been demonstrated by susceptibility testing, no further therapeutic benefit can be expected by continuing that drug. It follows that the prevalence of drug resistance is an index of the efficacy of antituberculosis chemotherapy within the community.

An important distinction has been made between the initial treatment and retreatment of patients with bacteriologically positive tuberculosis. It seems more important not to become overly involved in classifying patients as to whether or not they had received prior treatment but rather, whether or not the patient's tuberculous infection is susceptible or resistant to specific drugs. Nonetheless, it is true that patients who previously have received an effective course of chemotherapy and who had responded well, only to reactivate later, usually excrete tubercle bacilli susceptible to the drugs used in the original regimen. However, a variable percentage of relapsed patients have drug resistance and it is essential that a patient with any history of receiving antituberculosis chemotherapy have drug susceptibility tests performed. Therapy failure patients are those who have not responded satisfactorily to their chemotherapy and drug resistance is a frequent finding in such patients. The failure to complete an appropriate course of chemotherapy may be the result of inadequacies in the health care delivery system or of extremely difficult and demanding self-destructive characteristics of the individual tuberculosis patient.

The pathogenesis of drug resistance in therapy-failure patients is easily understood.[2] The tragic course of such a patient is demonstrated in Table 5. 1. Note that on 6/73, isoniazid and PAS therapy were begun in a patient whose bacteriologically positive pulmonary tuberculosis was fully susceptible to isoniazid, PAS, ethambutol and rifampin. As is so frequently the case in adults, the PAS was discontinued by the patient because of gastrointestinal side effects. It is not surprising that three months later, the patient's organisms are now resistant to isoniazid because he received, in effect, only one drug when the bacterial population was greatest and two drugs are necessary in such situations to ensure that bacterial resistance does not occur. At the 9/73 visit, a similar error is made by adding only one drug, ethambutol, to the failing regimen. The use of one drug in the presence of a large bacterial population of susceptible organisms or the addition of one drug to a failing regimen are the two most devastating mistakes possible in the management of tuberculosis. It is, therefore, not surprising that on 12/73, the only change has been the emergence of resistance to ethambutol. Once again the error is repeated and only rifampin is added to the failing regimen. As a result of rifampin's potency in eliminating susceptible organisms, a false sense of security is promoted on 2/74, because the bacterial population of susceptible organisms has been reduced sufficiently to achieve, albeit temporarily, a negative culture. However, by 4/74, the culture is again positive; and in 10 short months a patient who could have been adequately treated has been inflicted with an extremely difficult and potentially life-threatening situation. What remains for this unfortunate patient are less potent and much more toxic second line drugs.

TABLE 5.1

Drug	Date 6/73	9/73	12/73	2/74	4/74
INH	├────	────	────	────	────┤
PAS	├- - ? - -	- -┤			
Ethambutol		├────	────	────	────┤
Rifampin			├────	────	────┤
Culture	+	+	+	−	+
Drug susceptibility					
INH	S	R	R		R
PAS	S	S	S		S
Ethambutol	S	S	R		R
Rifampin	S	S	S		R

R = resistant   S = sensitive

The choice of the chemotherapeutic regimen for patients with drug resistant tuberculosis depnds upon the same principles that guide therapy for patients with susceptible organisms.[3] The problem is that the drugs available for such therapy usually are less effective and associated with more frequent and more severe side effects. The second line drugs are listed in Table II (Appendix 2). It is mandatory that an excellent bacteriology laboratory be available to identify the correct therapy for patients with resistant tuberculosis. If such facilities are not available, consultation should be obtained from the laboratories where such excellence is present. One strives for the institution of a chemotherapeutic regimen that contains at least two drugs to which the patient's tubercle bacilli are fully susceptible. At the beginning of therapy at least two, and preferably three drugs which the patient has not received are administered. Susceptibility tests should be available in one to two months and the clinican will also have the benefit of having followed the patient for that time. Signs that might be indicative of therapeutic effectiveness are an improvement in symptoms, a decrease in the number of organisms in the sputum smear, and some clearing of the chest x-ray. When the susceptibility tests are available, the regimen needs to be reexamined and a decision made as to whether or not the patient is receiving the most appropriate chemotherapy. Since so many of these patients are failures of an unsupervised, self-administered chemotherapy program, a supervised program of chemotherapy should be considered.

One of the simpler problems in the selection of a therapeutic regimen for drug resistant tuberculosis is for the patient whose tubercle bacilli are resistant to isoniazid but susceptible to ethambutol and rifampin. Clearly, the best choice is to administer the oral drugs ethambutol and rifampin. The addition of isoniazid in such a situation, advocated by some, seems not to be justified. Therapy usually is continued for twenty-four months after the patient with drug resistant disease demonstrates sputum culture negativity.

Much more difficult decisions must be made when confronted with resistance, either proven or suspected, to multiple first line drugs. In such a situation, one of the parenteral drugs most invariably must be used. The parenteral drugs, streptomycin, viomycin, kanamycin and capreomycin, are equally effective. However, because of a lower incidence of side effects, streptomycin is the first choice with kanamycin the second if resistance to streptomycin has been demonstrated or suspected because of previous administration. Each patient's chemotherapy for drug resistant tuberculosis must be carefully chosen and followed but the most frequently used regimens for such patients include capreomycin, rifampin, and pyrazinamide; capreomycin, ethiomanide, and pyrazinamide; and kanamycin, cycloserine, and pyrazinamide. Interestingly, while the necessity to discontinue one or more drugs of such three regimens may be as high as 30 percent, the addition of two to three more drugs, five or six in all, raises the discontinuation percentage to 40 percent.[1] However, this level of adverse drug reactions is very high and any opportunity to minimize this complication should be taken. The procedure to follow if second line drug toxicity is suspected is the same as when it is suspected with first line drugs: stop all medications and restart them one at a time, the least likely offender first, the most likely last.

CASE REPORT

RETREATMENT FOR RESISTANT DISEASE

The patient was born and lived in the Philippines until age 25 when she immigrated to the United States. She was well until May, 1973, when, at age 23, she experienced weight loss and fever. A chest x-ray film demonstrated bilateral cavities and the patient reportedly was treated with ethambutol and PAS until October, 1974, at which time she developed hemoptysis and changed physicians. Chest x-ray films were reported to her as worse, and her treatment was changed to isoniazid, rifampin, ethambutol and weekly injections of streptomycin. She received this regimen until she immigrated to the United States where it was continued until July, 1975. As far as can be determined, every sputum specimen that had been collected from May, 1973, to July, 1975, was smear and culture positive. Sensitivity tests were first performed on a sputum specimen obtained in March, 1975, and revealed partial resistance to isoniazid and cycloserine, full resistance to rifampin and sensitivity to ethambutol, PAS, streptomycin, viomycin and ethionamide.

A prolonged hospitalization was recommended in July, 1975, but the patient did not agree to start it until December, 1975. From July to December, 1975, she had been treated with isoniazid alone. At the time of hospitalization, she weighed 78 pounds and complained of a productive cough and occasional hemoptysis. A chest x-ray film (Figure 5.1) showed extensive bilateral cavitary disease with air fluid levels. A sputum culture obtained September, 1975, grew out catalase 3+ positive, niacin positive Mycobacterium tuberculosis. Indirect susceptibility tests revealed resistance to isoniazid, streptomycin, ethambutol, ethionamide and rifampin; the organism was sensitive

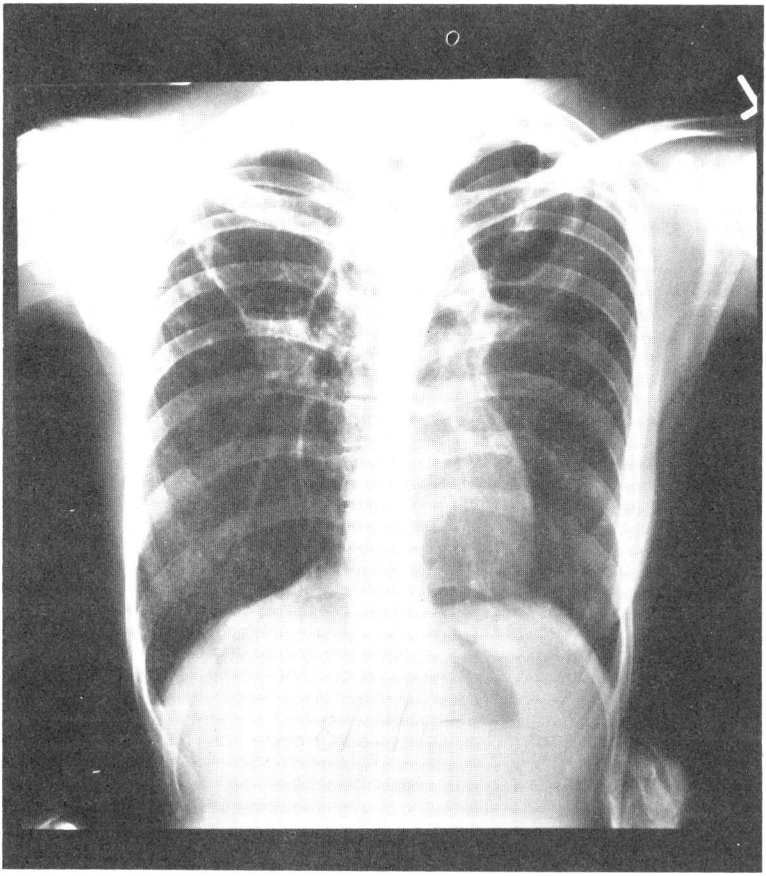

FIG. 5.1: Chest roentgenogram taken in August, 1975, of Case 1 revealing extensive bilateral infiltrates and cavitation with air-fluid levels.

to kanamycin, viomycin, capreomycin, high concentrations of PAS, pyrazinamide, and cycloserine. Admission sputum smears and cultures were all positive and direct sensitivity testing demonstrated sensitivity only to PAS, viomycin, cycloserine and capreomycin.

Therapy was initiated with pyrazinamide and viomycin on December 19 and cycloserine on December 28, 1975. On January 15, 1976, PAS was started but two days later the patient developed swelling of the ankles and bilateral knee effusions. Joint aspirations were sterile and antinuclear antibody and L. E. preparations were negative. It was felt that the knee effusions represented a drug reaction and all her medications were temporarily discontinued and subsequently restarted one by one. PAS was later discontinued because of nausea.

She was maintained on a regimen of pyrazinamide, 1.0 gm three times a day, viomycin 600 mg intramuscularly five days a week, cycloserine 250 mg three times per day, and pyridoxine hydrochloride 50 mg a day. She had profound swings in mood and the question of cycloserine toxicity was raised. The serum concentration of cycloserine while on 250 mg three times per day was determined at 33 mcg/ml two hours after a dose; the cycloserine was reduced to twice a day. On this regimen, the cycloserine level was 24 mcg/ml two hours after a dose. She demonstrated mild hyperuricemia, probably due to her pyrazinamide therapy, but no evidence of gout. Sputum smears were last positive on January 19, 1976, and the last positive culture on January 25, 1976. All subsequent smears and cultures were negative during her hospitalization and she was discharged in July, 1976.

She continued to do well as an outpatient. Her viomycin was discontinued in February, 1977, one year after her last positive sputum culture; and pyrazinamide and cycloserine were continued until February, 1978. She gained weight up to 98 pounds and her sputum smears and cultures have been consistently negative. Her chest x-ray films have demonstrated further improvement (Figure 5.2).

Comment: This patient demonstrates many of the problems frequently encountered in the treatment of a patient with drug-resistant tuberculosis. Whether or not the resistance is primary or secondary, the toxicity of the few available drugs, the emotional difficulties so often found in such patients, the necessity for prolonged hospitalizations, and the need for sophisticated laboratory resources capable of determining drug

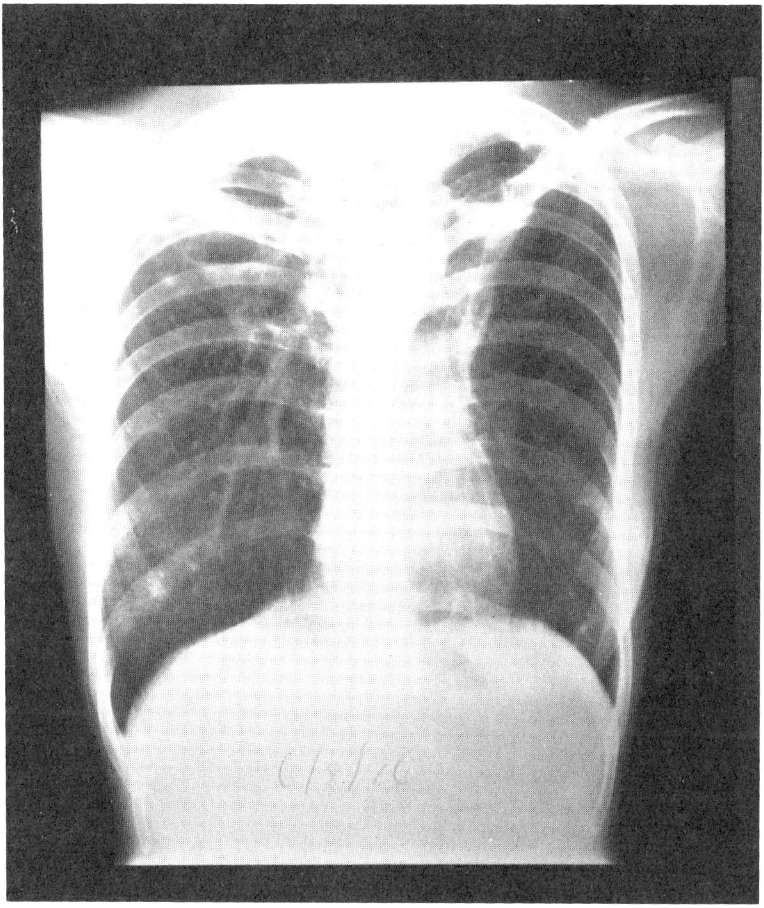

FIG. 5.2: Chest x-ray of Case 1 taken in June, 1976, revealing improvement of the bilateral pulmonary infiltrates and cavitation after six months of appropriate anti-tuberculous chemotherapy.

levels are all issues that must be faced with these patients. This patient also demonstrates that if these problems are solved, chemotherapy can be successfully completed. In this woman, the hospitalization period was beautifully managed at The National Jewish Hospital in Denver, Colorado.

REFERENCES

1. Lester W: Treatment of Drug-Resistant Tuberculosis. Disease-A-Month. Year Book Publishers. April, 1971.

2. Cheung OT: Drug-resistant pulmonary tuberculosis. Am Rev Resp Dis 111:900, 1976.

3. Branscomb BV, Lester W, McDonald TM, et al.: Chemotherapy of pulmonary tuberculosis: The choice of drugs in relation to drug susceptibility. Am Rev Resp Dis 92:2, 1965.

CHAPTER VI:

THE MYCOBACTERIOSES

There are several mycobacteria, other than M. tuberculosis, which produce disease in man. Before the effective control of M. bovis disease in cattle and pasteurization of milk, infection with this organism was quite common in human beings; however, it is now rare.

Several atypical mycobacteria may cause human disease. Although these organisms have constituted a small proportion of the total number of cases of tuberculosis in the past, as clinical M. tuberculosis infections continue to decrease in incidence, their relative importance will increase.

The group of organisms to which we are now referring have been termed "Unclassified Mycobacteria", "Anonymous Mycobacteria" and "Atypical Mycobacteria". The term "atypical tuberculosis" has been widely used to describe the diseases produced by these organisms. There is, however, no general agreement on a title for this group of diseases. We prefer the term "Mycobacterioses".

In 1959, Runyon classified these organisms into four groups on the basis of their pigmentary and growth characteristics.[1] They are generally cultured much more rapidly in the laboratory than other mycobacteria, and the fourth classification in the group, the "Rapid Growers", is usually recovered in one week. The first group in the Runyon classification, the "Photochromogenic" organisms, produce a typical yellow pigment when grown in the light. The second group, the "Scotochromogens", produce pigment when grown in the dark. The third group in the Runyon classification consists of the "Nonchromogenic" organisms.

The fact that these organisms do not produce progressive granulomatous disease in guinea pigs is thought to have delayed their recognition and acceptance as a pathogen for man. The refinement of culture methods and newer, less harsh digestive procedures have led to an increasing rate of recovery and identification of these organisms.

It has been suggested that there is a significant association between chronic lung diseases, such as the pneumoconioses and the chronic obstructive lung diseases, and infection with atypical mycobacteria. In many cases, however, no antecedent pulmonary disease can be documented. These diseases do not appear to be communicable.

GROUP I

The most common pathogenic photochromogenic organisms are M. kansasii and M. marinum. The former produces pulmonary disease, and the latter, superficial skin lesions or abscesses with nodules and nodes in the distribution of lymphatic drainage. Skin lesions secondary to M. marinum usually arise from contact with swimming pools and small, domestic fish tanks.

M. kansasii produces pulmonary disease which histologically resembles M. tuberculosis. The chest roentgenogram is frequently not distinguishable from disease secondary to M. tuberculosis. Occasionally, a thin-walled solitary cavity with very little surrounding infiltrate may be seen (Figure 6.1). This roentgenographic appearance simulates the classic single, thin-walled cavity frequently seen in coccidioidomycosis infection of the lung.

M. kansasii pulmonary infection may be seen anywhere in the United States, but most patients have been reported in the Midwest and Southwest. The diagnosis is made on the basis of cultures of sputum, tissue, tissue aspirates or body fluids. Once the diagnosis has been established, the treatment has traditionally consisted of triple drug therapy with isoniazid, ethambutol, and either streptomycin or rifampin. Recently, many authorities have considered a combination of INH and rifampin equally effective. These patients respond well to chemotherapy despite variable degrees of drug resistance in vitro, and surgical intervention is rarely required.[2, 3] A combined chemotherapeutic and surgical approach was frequently used several years ago. Subsequent excellent experience with drug therapy alone has led us to avoid surgery for these patients. It has been our custom to treat these patients with triple drug chemotherapy for a total of twenty-four months. The incidence of relapse after cessation of chemotherapy appears to be greater than with M. tuberculosis, and regular follow-up evaluation is indicated in patients who have

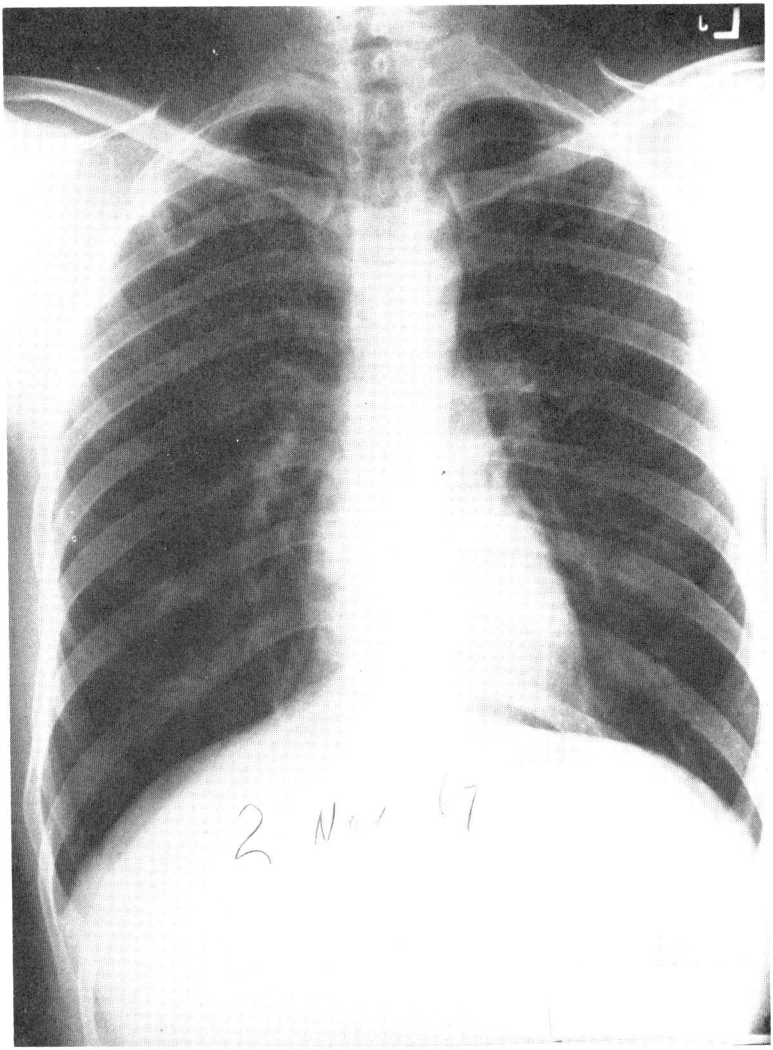

FIG. 6.1: Thin-walled cavity in the right upper lobe, with minimal surrounding infiltrate, resulting from M. kansasii infection.

been treated for M. kansasii disease. Relapse is usually easily managed by reinstitution of chemotherapy or the addition of rifampin to the previous regimen.

GROUP II

Pulmonary disease due to M. scrofulaceum is extremely rare. Recovery of scotochromogens from sputum is usually of no significance and the interpretation of repeated isolation of these organisms from a patient with a pulmonary infiltrate must be approached with caution.[4] A form of chronic lymphadenitis resembling classic scrofula is seen in children and adolescents in which the causative organism is M. scrofulaceum. The treatment of this condition usually involves a combined surgical and chemotherapeutic approach.

GROUP III

The nonchromogenic mycobacteria of clinical significance includes M. intracellulare (Battey bacillus), M. avium, M. ulcerans and M. xenopi. Human disease due to M. avium and M. xenopi is rare. M. intracellulare, however, is a frequent cause of an indolent, progressive, pulmonary disease radiologically similar to M. tuberculosis. Recently, the term Avium Complex or Avium-intracellulare Complex has been adopted to describe M. intracellulare and M. avium as one group of organisms.

The original reports of clinical M. intracellulare infection were from the southeastern United States.[5] Subsequent reports have shown, however, that this infection is a significant problem elsewhere.[2, 6, 7] Skin tests performed with antigen obtained from M. intracellulare have been shown to produce a positive delayed hypersensitivity reaction in a large proportion of the population in Georgia. In addition, the organism has been isolated from sputum and throat cultures obtained from healthy persons and from the soil in the same area. It would appear that the organism is acquired from the environment, is of low virulence and is not communicable. This statement regarding communicability holds true for all of the atypical mycobacteria.[8]

M. intracellulare pulmonary infection is an extremely vexing problem because as many as five simultaneous antituberculous drugs may infrequently be required to adequately control the infection. Adverse drug reactions are extremely common with the use of so many drugs, and patient compliance is frequently poor. Some patients, however, appear to respond to conventional three-drug therapy.

It has been suggested that, when treating localized disease secondary to M. intracellulare, the best therapy is surgical resection after a period of adequate chemotherapy[5] (Figures 6.2 and 6.3). On the other hand, it has also been suggested that resection rarely removes all of the organisms. Many patients have advanced bilateral disease and are not surgical candidates (Figure 6.4). In one study, seventeen of eighteen patients undergoing lobectomy after a six-month trial of chemotherapy had a good result including bacteriologic remission. However, six patients subsequently experienced bacteriologic relapse.[7]

Of all of the mycobacterial infections, M. intracellulare is the most difficult to treat successfully. Unless one is experienced in the therapy of this disease, expert consultation should be obtained before medical or surgical therapy is instituted. M. intracellulare may also be recovered from sputum in the absence of infection and it is important to correlate the chest roentgenogram and clinical finding with the culture results.

GROUP IV

"Rapid growers" have been reported to produce cervical adenitis, self-limited pneumonitis and "cold abscesses", osteomyelitis and miliary disease in the immunosuppressed host. The major pathogens in this group are the M. fortuitum - M. abscessus group. In our experience, these organisms only rarely produce clinical disease.

SKIN TESTS FOR ATYPICAL ORGANISMS

Skin test antigen is available for M. kansaii, M. scrofulaceum and M. intracellulare; these have been used widely in epidemiologic studies. Unfortunately, these specific skin tests are of little value in the individual patient. The intermediate PPD skin test is frequently negative in active M. kansasii and Avium-Complex infection, while the second strength PPD (250 TU) is positive. Although of interest, differential reactions of the various atypical antigens in comparison with Tween 80 stabilized PPD intermediate (5 TU) are not diagnostic. Only through culture and identification of the organism can the diagnosis of atypical tuberculosis be substantiated.

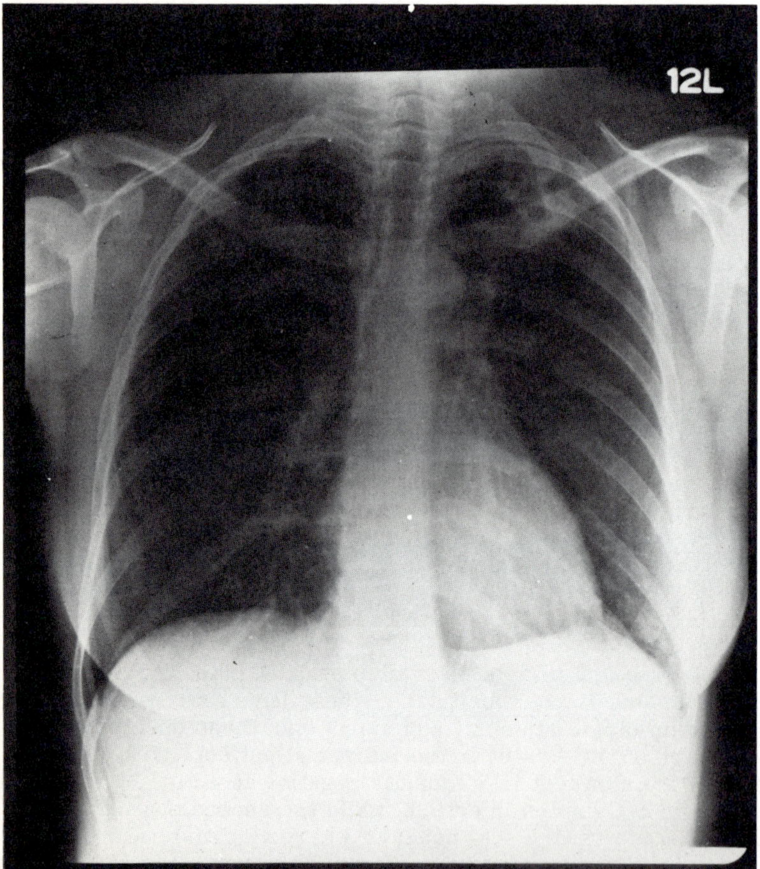

FIG. 6.2: Cavitating infiltrate in the left upper lobe secondary to M. intracellulare infection.

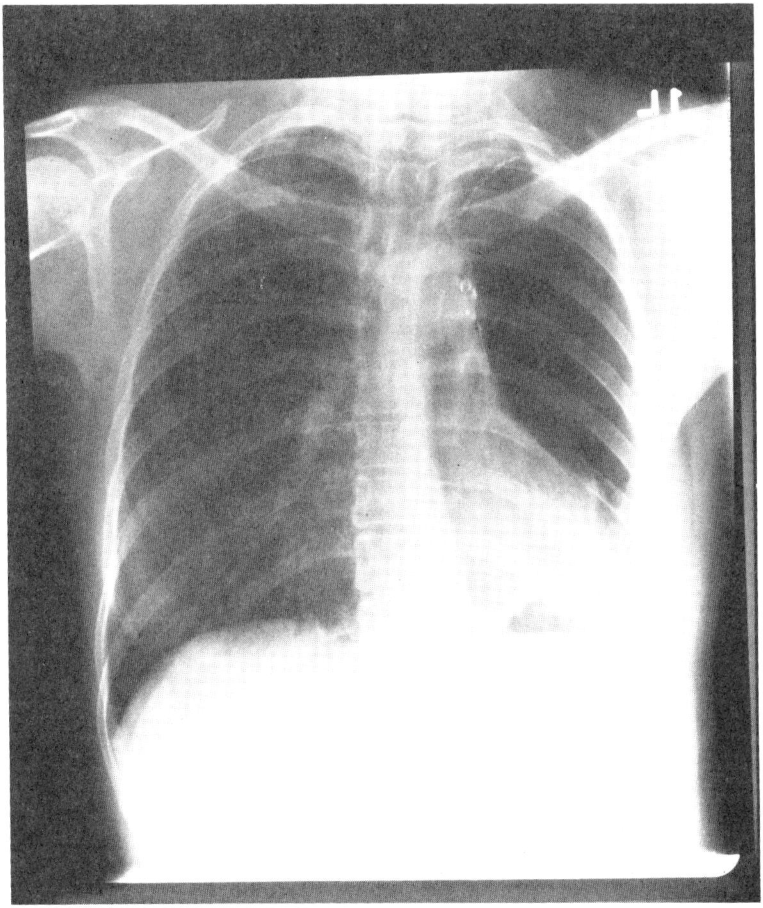

FIG. 6.3: Chest roentgenogram of patient shown in Fig. 6.2, following resection of disease in left upper lobe.

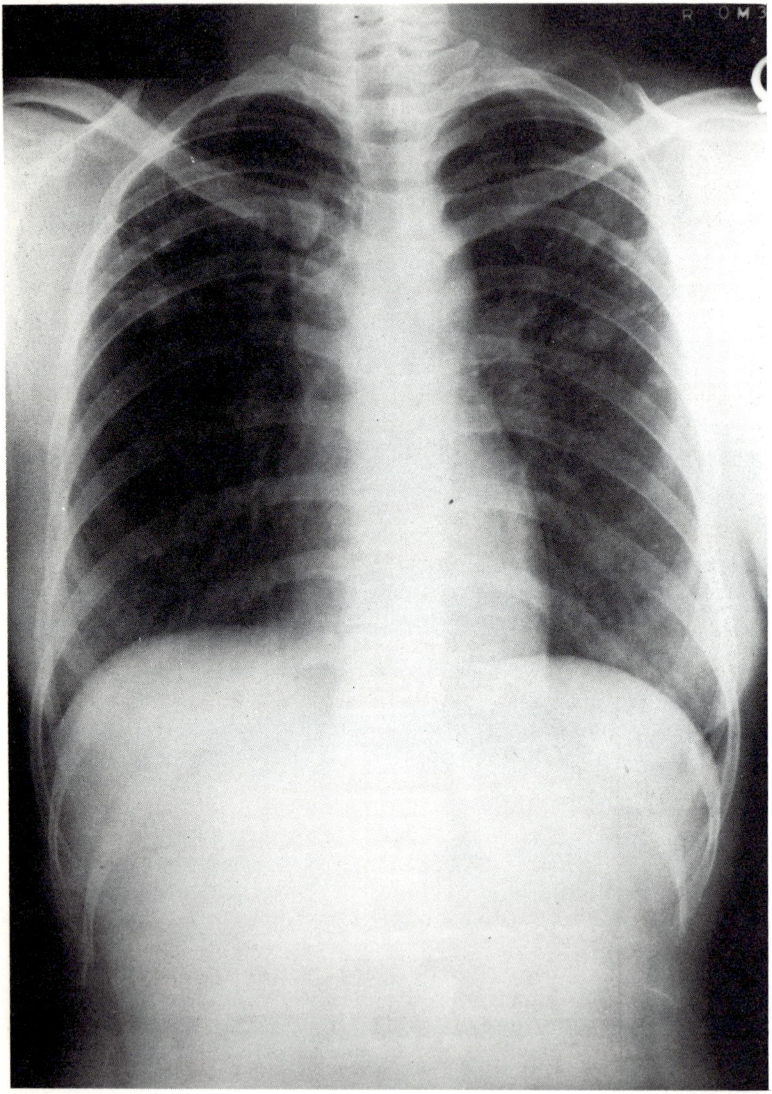

FIG. 6.4: Extensive bilateral fibronodular disease resulting from M. intracellulare infection.

ILLUSTRATIVE CASES

CASE 1: PRIMARY TREATMENT

A 48-year-old Caucasian male assembly-line worker presented for evaluation of an abnormal routine chest roentgenogram (Figure 6.5). He denied significant symptoms. On direct questioning he admitted to a chronic, minimally productive cough.

The physical examination and routine laboratory evaluation were both unremarkable. Three spontaneous sputum specimens were positive on smear for AFB. The PPD intermediate skin test (5 TU) was negative. The second PPD (250 TU) was positive with 15 mm of induration.

The patient was placed on triple antituberculous chemotherapy consisting of isoniazid, 300 mg once daily; ethambutol, 25 mg/kg once daily; and rifampin, 600 mg once daily. Subsequently, sputum cultures were all positive for M. kansasii.

After ninety days of antituberculous chemotherapy, the sputum AFB stain became negative and the chest roentgenogram revealed definitive improvement. A few organisms were still obtained on culture. All subsequent AFB smears and cultures were negative. Over the next twelve months, the infiltrate on the chest roentgenogram cleared completely. Treatment was continued for a total of twenty-four months and then discontinued. Subsequent chest roentgenograms have remained unremarkable.

Comment: This patient responded well to triple antituberculous chemotherapy. Rifampin was used instead of streptomycin, because patients find this drug more acceptable than long-term injections. In addition, it is frequently difficult to arrange convenient long-term parenteral drug therapy for outpatients. Lester and associates found that 100% of patients with disease secondary to M. kansasii responded to initial chemotherapy.[2] In addition, thirty-four of thirty-five patients with M. kansasii infection achieved quiescent status on retreatment.[3] In our experience, disease secondary to M. kansasii responds excellently to triple-drug chemotherapy and surgery is rarely indicated.

CASE 2: PRIMARY TREATMENT

A 44-year-old male was found to have an abnormal chest roentgenogram on a routine pre-employment examination

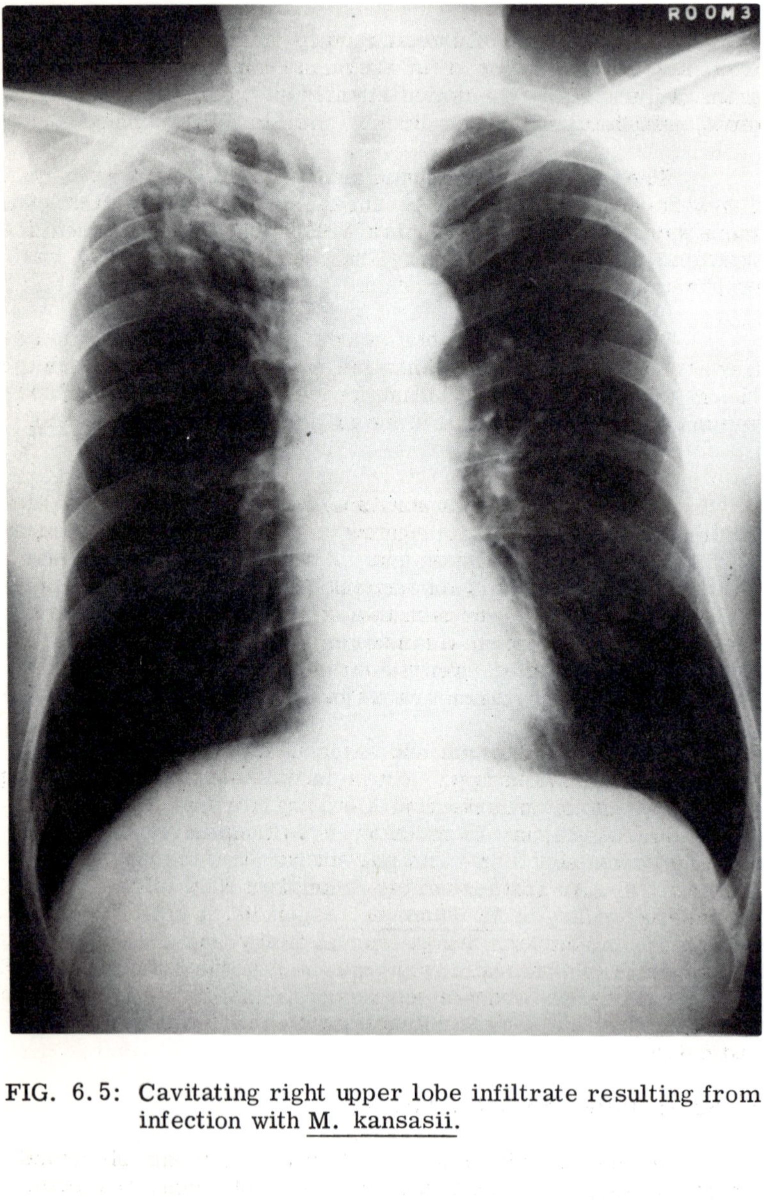

FIG. 6.5: Cavitating right upper lobe infiltrate resulting from infection with M. kansasii.

(Figure 6. 6). He was asymptomatic except for a chronic "cigarette cough". The physical examination was entirely unremarkable.

Review of several prior chest roentgenograms, obtained while the patient was in the military service, revealed that he had had progressive bilateral pulmonary infiltrates for at least four years.

Skin tests with several antigens revealed: negative Tween 80 stabilized intermediate PPD (5 TU); PPD-Battey (PPD-B) 7 mm induration; and Second Strength PPD (250 TU) - 38 mm induration. Sputum smears were markedly positive for acid-fast bacilli.

Antituberculous chemotherapy was instituted consisting of isoniazid, 300 mg daily; streptomycin, one gram daily; and ethambutol, 15 mg/kg/day. Three weeks later, it was confirmed that the patient's sputum cultures were positive for nonpigmented atypical organisms. Subsequent identification revealed that these organisms were M. intracellulare. Drug sensitivity studies revealed resistance, in vitro, to all first and second line drugs. At this point, rifampin, 600 mg/day; ethionamide, one gram daily; and pyrazinamide, 2. 5 grams daily were added to his drug therapy for a total of six drugs. In addition, the isoniazid was increased to 600 mg daily and ethambutol to 25 mg/kg/day. Pyridoxine hydrochloride was added to his drug regimen because of the high isoniazid dose.

Six weeks after the initiation of drug therapy, the streptomycin dose was reduced to one gram three times a week. The patient had begun to note occasional slight tinnitus at this point in time. In addition, the patient noted some moderate but tolerable gastrointestinal intolerance as a result of the ethionamide.

Eight weeks after chemotherapy was started, the patient began to note vague arthralgias primarily in the knees, ankles, and proximal interphalangeal joints of the hands with some stiffness. There were no objective joint changes and the serum uric acid remained normal. It was suspected that either the isoniazid or pyrazinamide were producing these symptoms. All drug therapy was discontinued for two weeks with no change noted in the arthralgias. The chemotherapy was restarted.

The patient remained culture negative from the fourth month of chemotherapy, for the full twenty-four months of chemotherapy. However, although there was some improvement in

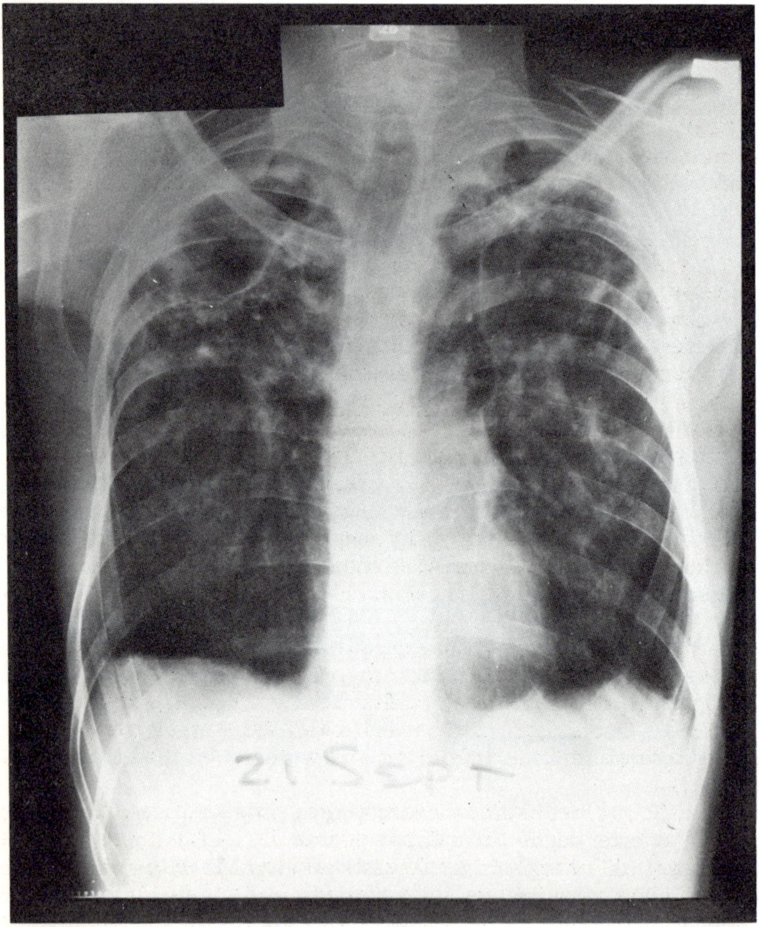

FIG. 6.6: Extensive bilateral M. intracellulare infection with fibronodular changes, bilateral cavitation and pleural thickening.

the chest roentgenograms after twenty-four months of therapy, significant residual disease remained bilaterally (Figure 6. 7).

The patient developed progressive rheumatoid arthritis with deformity of the hands during therapy which was not proven to be related to the drug therapy. Pyrazinamide was eventually discontinued as it could not be ascertained that the arthritis was unrelated to the use of this drug. In addition, late in the course of therapy, the patient developed symptoms and signs of a peripheral neuropathy which was suspected, but not proven, to be related to the use of isoniazid. It should be noted that the patient was being given supplemental pyridoxine throughout the course of this chemotherapy.

Comment: This patient is an excellent example of the problems and frustrations frequently involved in the treatment of Group III, M. intracellulare, infection. The patient did respond to chemotherapy and converted to a culture-negative status. Many patients do not respond, even to multiple drug therapy. On the other hand, rare patients with M. intracellulare infection respond to conventional three-drug therapy, despite apparent drug resistance on in vitro testing. Certain patients with localized M. intracellulare disease might be considered for combination chemotherapy and surgical resection. This patient, with extensive bilateral disease, was certainly not a surgical candidate. Surgical resection for localized disease secondary to M. intracellulare seems logical. However, Rosenzweig found that of eighteen patients undergoing lobectomy for localized M. intracellulare infection, one remained bacteriologically positive postoperatively and six patients subsequently relapsed.[7]

This patient illustrates another problem seen in patients who are receiving multiple drug therapy--that of adverse drug reaction. This patient developed tinnitus as a result of streptomycin, mild gastrointestinal disturbance from ethionamide, and a peripheral neuropathy which may have been isoniazid-related. Deforming rheumatoid arthritis was also initially suspected but not proven to be related to pyrazinamide. Multiple drug therapy of this type is almost invariably associated with adverse reactions, some of which may be lethal. Frequently, adverse gastrointestinal, systemic, and vestibular reactions will lead patients to discontinue all or part of their chemotherapeutic program. In our opinion, the proper approach to the treatment of M. intracellulare infection has not been defined at this point in time. It has even been suggested that perhaps no treatment is in order in light of the indolent nature of this disease unless the

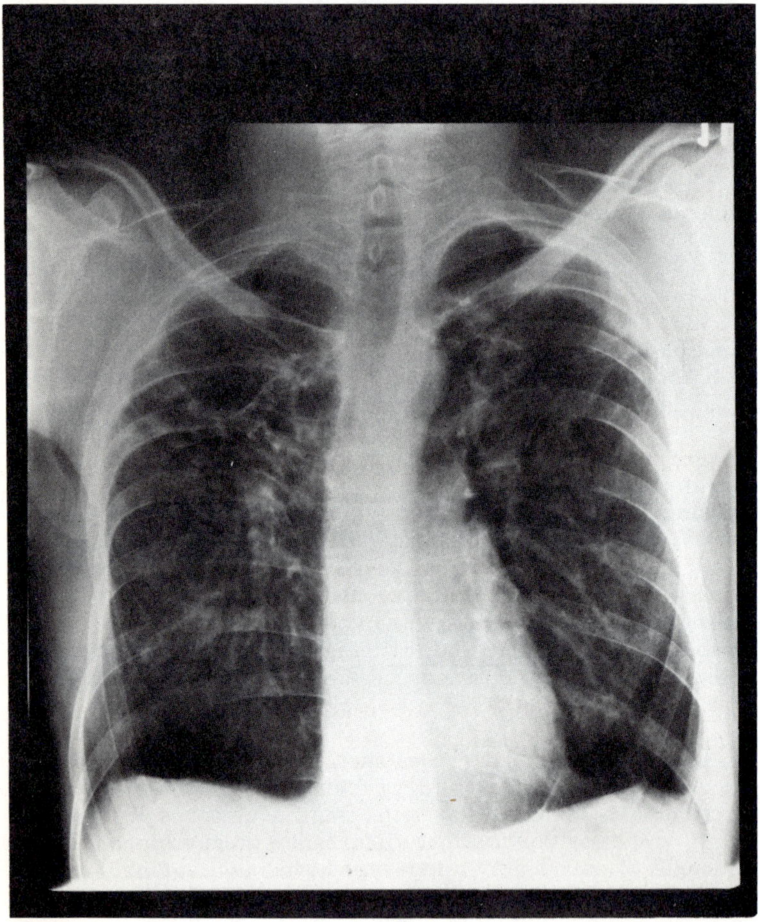

FIG. 6.7: Chest roentgenogram of patient shown in Fig. 6.6 following twenty-four months of antituberculous chemotherapy, revealing extensive bilateral residual changes. Sputum cultures for M. intracellulare had been persistently negative for eighteen months at the time that this roentgenogram was obtained.

patient is symptomatic. A national cooperative study is needed to help resolve this problem.

CASE 3: PRIMARY TREATMENT

A 76-year-old retired businessman presented for a routine physical examination. His only complaint was poor eyesight. He denied pulmonary symptoms.

The routine chest roentgenogram revealed a small area of segmental, finely nodular infiltrate, in the left lower lobe (Figures 6.8 and 6.9). Review of a chest roentgenogram taken one year previously revealed that the infiltrate had not been present at that time. Fungal serologies were negative. Three induced sputa obtained for cytology were negative for malignant cells. Three induced sputum specimens followed by gastric washings were obtained for mycobacterial and fungal studies. Smears for AFB were negative.

The patient's PPD intermediate skin test (5 TU) was positive, with 10 mm induration. The patient was placed on isoniazid, 300 mg daily; and ethambutol, 25 mg/kg/day, pending the result of cultures. Subsequently, two sputa and two gastric washings grew out nonchromogenic atypical mycobacteria, "a few colonies". These organisms were identified as M. intracellulare. Drug sensitivity studies revealed complete resistance to isoniazid, PAS, streptomycin, ethambutol, viomycin, rifampin, and cycloserine.

Three months after institution of chemotherapy with isoniazid and ethambutol, the chest roentgenogram revealed complete clearing of the infiltrate. The one induced sputum obtained at that time was negative on AFB smear. The culture subsequently grew out one colony of M. intracellulare. Antituberculous chemotherapy was continued with isoniazid and ethambutol (15 mg/kg/day) for a total of eighteen months. The chest roentgenogram remained negative.

Comment: This patient exhibits the problem which frequently arises when Group II (Scotochromogens) and Group III (Avium-Complex, M. intracellulare) organisms are isolated from sputum and gastric washings. These organisms are frequently saprophytic and of no clinical significance when isolated. However, the decision as to their clinical importance may be extremely difficult to make. The appearance of the current and prior chest roentgenogram, clinical course, and source of the positive culture must all be considered before assuming that the

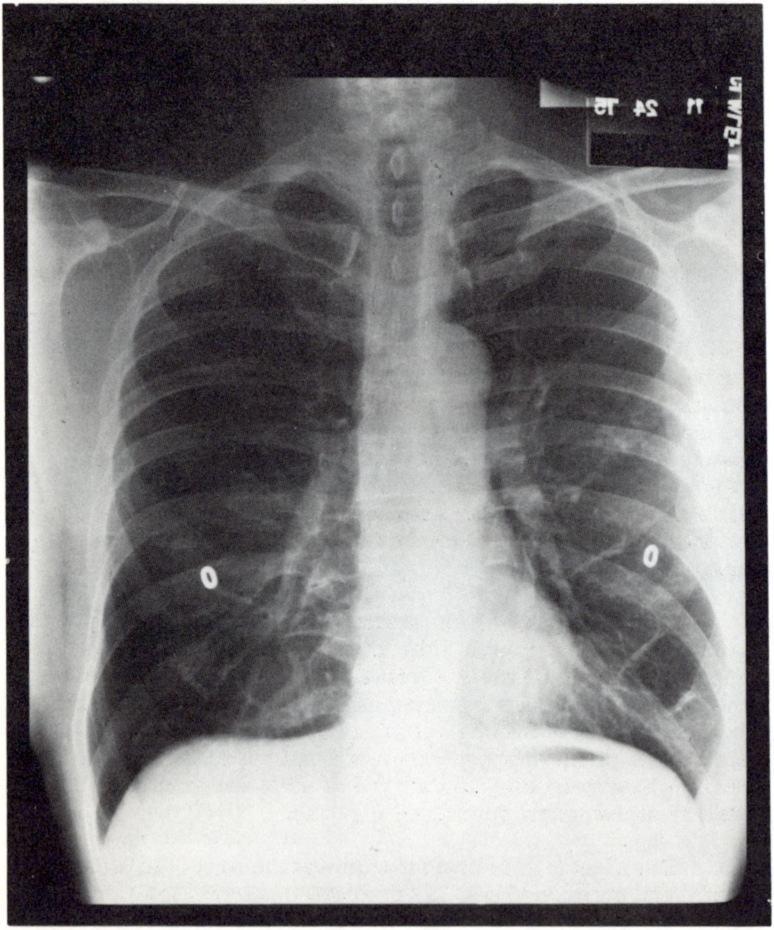

FIG. 6.8: Small area of fibronodular infiltrate in the posterior aspect of the left upper lobe.

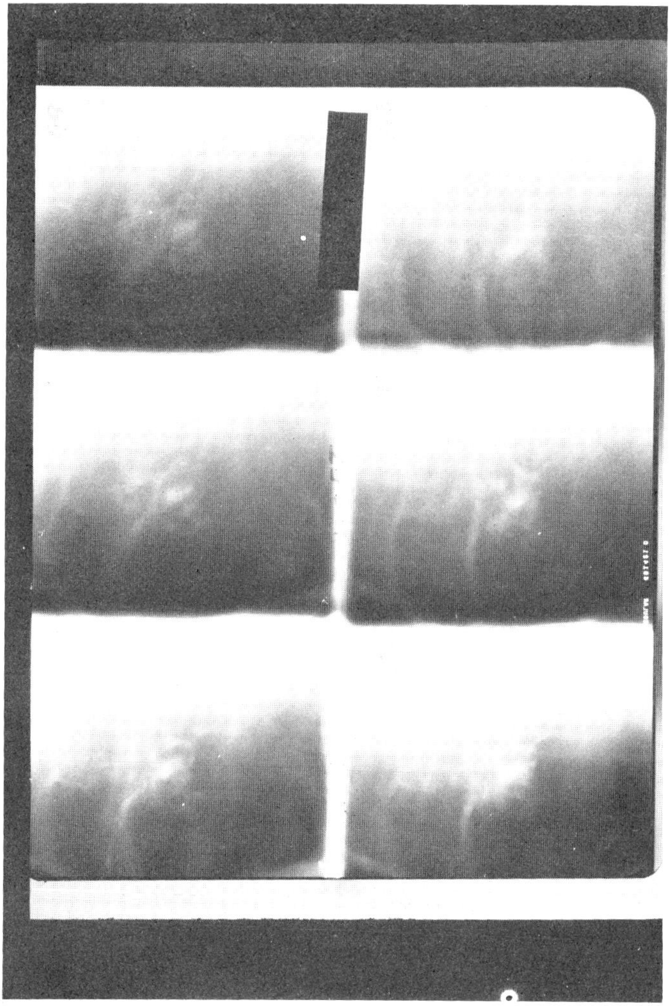

FIG. 6.9: Tomograms of the left upper lobe infiltrate noted in Fig. 6.8.

isolation of these organisms is clinically significant.[4]

The patient described cleared the infiltrate rapidly while on antituberculous chemotherapy. Whether the infiltrate was tuberculous, M. tuberculosis or M. intracellulare, is not certain. It did resolve while on treatment. In light of the clearing on the chest roentgenogram and positive PPD skin test, we felt that we had no choice but to continue the isoniazid and ethambutol for a total of 18 months. To us, it seems unlikely that this was an infection resulting from M. intracellulare.

REFERENCES

1. Runyon, E. H.: Anonymous mycobacteria in pulmonary disease. Med Clin North Am 43:273-290, 1959.

2. Lester, W., Carnright, L., et al.: Results of antituberculosis chemotherapy in 130 cases of disease by atypical mycobacteria. Cincinnati, Ohio. Trans 30th Res Conf Pulm Dis, January, 1971, p. 44.

3. Harris, G. D., Johnason, W. G., Jr., and Nicholson, D.: Response to chemotherapy of pulmonary infection due to Mycobacterium kansasii. Bulletin of the Int. Union Against Tuberculosis, Vol. 2, No. 1, Tome 1:275, 1976.

4. Gracey, D. R., Byrd, R. B.: Scotochromogens and pulmonary disease. Am Rev Respir Dis 101:959, 1970.

5. Corpe, R. F.: Clinical aspects, medical and surgical, in the management of Battey-type pulmonary disease. Dis Chest 45:380, 1964.

6. Edwards, F. G. B.: Disease caused by "atypical" (opportunistic) mycobacteria: A whole population review. Tubercle 51:285, 1970.

7. Rosenzweig, D. Y.: Course and long-term follow-up of 100 cases of pulmonary infection due to M. avium intercellulare complex (M. a-i). Am Rev Respir Dis 113:(Suppl) 55, 1976.

8. Girard, W. M., Ahn, D. H., Light, R. W., Cush, R., Goerge, R. B.: Epidemiology of atypical mycobacterial disease in Texas and Louisiana. Bulletin of the Int. Union Against Tuberculosis, Vol. 2, No. 1, Tome 1:263, 1976.

CHAPTER VII:

SURGICAL THERAPY OF PULMONARY TUBERCULOSIS

Prior to the availability of antituberculous chemotherapy, surgery played a major role in the treatment of pulmonary tuberculosis. Extraperiosteal paravertebral thoracoplasty, plombage thoracoplasty and resectional therapy were widely employed for active pulmonary tuberculosis prior to the introduction of effective chemotherapeutic agents. Subsequent to the development of adequate chemotherapeutic programs, resectional surgery continued to be used as a frequent adjunct to chemotherapy. However, as greater experience and more effective chemotherapeutic programs have been obtained, the indications for surgery have rapidly diminished. At the present time, surgical intervention is rarely needed. An occasional patient may require resection, thoracoplasty and resection or extrapleural pneumonectomy. In our experience, the indications for surgery are very few.

The indications for surgery in pulmonary tuberculosis fall into three general categories--punitive, relative, and definite.[1] Unstable and unrelaible patients such as alcoholics, drug addicts and sociopaths, who may constitute a hazard to society, are frequently subjected to surgical procedures when more conservative methods of treatment fail. In general, the problem in managing these patients has been the inflexible attitude of the program or physician dealing with the patient. Adequate chemotherapeutic programs often can be instituted which are acceptable to these problem patients utilizing innovative outpatient care.[2, 3] Chemotherapeutic failure in the unreliable patient frequently is a failure of the health care delivery system to meet the special needs and problems of the patient. Although the occasional patient may be considered for surgical resection on the basis of persistent positive sputum and residual disease, one must always question whether the patient is taking his chemotherapy regularly and evaluate for drug-resistant disease.

The relative indications for surgery include a totally destoyed lobe or lung, chronic empyema with or without bronchopleural fistula, chronic lower lobe cavitation, and bronchiectasis. Symptoms, the chemotherapeutic history, and other factors peculiar to the individual patient must be weighed in making a decision about surgery in these patients.

The absolute indications for surgery include: tuberculous bronchostenosis; symptomatic, culture negative, localized tuberculous bronchiectasis despite an adequate medical program; and massive uncontrollable and life-threatening hemoptysis.

Although resection was formerly widely used for the treatment of patients with residual cavity and negative cultures (the open negative cavity), this is no longer felt to be an indication for surgery. The status of the patient with localized disease secondary to drug resistant M. tuberculosis and M. intracellulare, not responding to chemotherapy, remains an unresolved problem from the surgical standpoint. Although some advocate resection of these patients in an attempt to eradicate the disease, others suggest that it is improbable that surgical resection removes all of the organisms and that residual disease will likely recur.[4]

In summary, surgical intervention is rarely required in the treatment of pulmonary tuberculosis today. In most cases, failure of drug therapy can be explained on the basis of drug resistance or poor patient compliance. Both of these situations can be corrected by the proper chemotherapeutic program. The approach to the patient with punitive or relative indications for surgery must be highly individualized. The absolute indications for surgery in tuberculosis are less controversial but in these situations, the therapy must also be individualized. The presence and severity of coexisting medical problems must be considered. If, for example, the patient has chronic obstructive lung disease, complete pulmonary physiologic studies must be performed before submitting the patient to surgery.

REFERENCES

1. Shields TW, Lees WM, Fox RT: Pulmonary tuberculosis and other mycobacterial infections of the lung. General Thoracic Surgery Lea and Febiger, Philadelphia, 1972.

2. American Thoracic Society: Intermittent therapy for adults with tuberculosis. Am Rev Respir Dis 110:374, 1974.

3. Fox W, Mitchison DA: Short course chemotherapy for pulmonary tuberculosis. Am Rev Respir Dis 111:845, 1975.

4. Rosenzweig DY: Course and long-term follow-up of 100 cases of pulmonary infection due to M. avium intracellulare complex (Ma-i) Am Rev Respir Dis 113:(Suppl) 55, 1976.

APPENDICES

APPENDIX 1

TABLE I

CLASSIFICATION OF TUBERCULOSIS*

O: No tuberculosis exposure, not infected (no history of exposure, negative tuberculin skin test)

I: Tuberculosis exposure, no evidence of infection (history of exposure, negative tuberculin skin test)

II: Tuberculous infection, without disease (positive tuberculin skin test, negative bacteriological studies (if done), no roentgenogram findings compatible with tuberculosis, no symptoms due to tuberculosis)

Chemotherapy status (preventive therapy):

A. None
B. On chemotherapy since (date)
C. Chemotherapy terminated (date)

1. Complete (prescribed course of therapy)
2. Incomplete

III: Tuberculosis: infected, with disease

A. Location of Disease (predominant site; other sites if significant)

1. Pulmonary
2. Pleural
3. Lymphatic
4. Bone or joint
5. Genitourinary
6. Miliary
7. Meningeal
8. Peritoneal
9. Other

*Summarized from Diagnostic Standards and Classification of Tuberculosis and Other Mycobacterial Diseases. American Lung Association, New York, 1974.

B. Bacteriological Status

1. Positive by:
   a) Microscopy only (date)
   b) Culture only (date)
   c) Microscopy and culture (date)

2. Negative (date)
3. Pending
4. Not done

C. Chemotherapy Status

1. None
2. On chemotherapy since (date)
3. Chemotherapy terminated (date)
   a) Complete (prescribed course of therapy)
   b) Incomplete

The following data are necessary in certain circumstances:

D. Roentgenogram Findings

1. Normal
2. Abnormal
   a) Cavitary or noncavitary
   b) Stable or worsening or improving

E. Tuberculin Skin Test

1. Positive reaction
2. Doubtful reaction
3. Negative reaction
4. Not done

Tuberculosis suspect: may be used until diagnostic procedures are complete but not for more than three months.

CLASSIFICATION OF OTHER MYCOBACTERIAL DISEASES

Mycobacterial disease caused by (name of organism)

A. Location of disease (predominant site; other sites if significant)

1. Pulmonary

2. Pleural
3. Lymphatic
4. Bone or joint
5. Genitourinary
6. Miliary
7. Meningeal
8. Peritoneal
9. Other

B. Bacteriological Status (species name when known or Runyon's classification until species name is known)

1. Positive by
   a) Culture only (date)
   b) Microscopy and culture (date)

2) Negative
3) Pending

C. Chemotherapy Status

1. None
2. On chemotherapy since (date)
3. Chemotherapy terminated (date)
   a) Complete (prescribed course of therapy)
   b) Incomplete

D. Roentgenogram Findings (useful in certain circumstances)

1. Normal
2. Abnormal
   a) Cavitary or noncavitary
   b) Stable or worsening or improving

APPENDIX 2

TABLE II

DOSES AND CHARACTERISTICS OF ANTITUBERCULOUS DRUGS

DRUG	DOSE	SIDE EFFECTS	MONITORING	REMARKS	SITE OF ACTION
Isoniazid	300 mg single daily dose (adult)	Peripheral Neuritis		Pyridoxine: 10 mg for prophylaxis; 50 mg to 100 mg for treatment	DNA Synthesis (Bacteriocidal)
		Hepatitis	SGOT, SGPT (if symptomatic)	Discontinue if symptomatic +/or liver enzymes more than twice normal	

		Central Nervous System: convulsions, optic neuritis with atrophy muscle twitching, dizziness, ataxia, toxic encephalopathy	CNS side effects are rare and cease after discontinuation of isoniazid	
		Hypersensitivity-- fever, rash	Rare; discontinue	
		Hematopoietic	Rare	
		Pyridoxine responsive anemia	Pyridoxine	
		?agranulocytosis	Discontinue	
		?aplastic anemia	Discontinue	
		Rheumatic and drug-induced lupus syndromes	Rare; discontinue	
		Dilantin toxicity	Reduce Dilantin	Delayed excretion
Rifampin	600 mg sin- single daily dose (adult)	Orange urine, tears, saliva	Reassure patient	RNA Syn- thesis (Bacter- iocidal) (cont'd.)

DRUG	DOSE	SIDE EFFECTS	MONITORING	REMARKS	SITE OF ACTION
Rifampin (cont'd.)		Flu-like syndrome		Need not discontinue rifampin and may restart if do discontinue	
		Hepatitis	SGOT, SGPT (if symptomatic)	Discontinue if jaundiced and/or liver enzymes more than twice normal	
		Thrombocytopenia	Platelet count	Anti-rifampin antibodies absorbed on platelets, fix complement, results in platelet damage; discontinue rifampin	
		Hemolysis		Drug related antibody fixes and activates complement; discontinue (? with intermittent therapy only)	
		Renal failure		Probably on immunological basis	

Drug Interactions:		
Warfarin	Protime	Rifampin decreases the hypoprothrombinemic effect of warfarin; warfarin dose may need to be reduced when rifampin discontinued
Oral contraceptives		Pregnancy reported in women on rifampin and oral contraceptives which may have accelerated catabolism caused by enzyme induction
Methadone		Rifampin may be associated with withdrawal symptoms in patients on a methadone maintenance program; also probably related to accelerated catabolism caused by enzyme induction

(cont'd.)

DRUG	DOSE	SIDE EFFECTS	MONITORING	REMARKS	SITE OF ACTION
		P.A.S.		Concomitant administration of PAS and rifampin may lead to decreased absorption of rifampin	
		Leukopenia	Leukocyte count	Rare	
Ethambutol	25 mg/kg in one daily dose for 2 weeks, then 15 mg/kg in on dose daily	Optic Neuritis	Visual acuity and red-green color discrimination	Rare at 15 mg/kg dose; more common at 25 mg/kg; use with caution in presence of renal insufficiency	RNA Synthesis (Bacteriostatic)
Para-amino salicylic acid (sodium salt)	200 mg/kg/day in 3 divided doses	Gastrointestinal--anorexia, nausea		Gastrointestinal intolerance extremely common in adult, less so in children	Intermediary metabolism (Bacteriostatic)
		Hypersensitivity reactions: fever, rash, arthritis		Discontinue	

		Hepatotoxicity	SGOT, SGPT	Discontinue	
		Sodium Load		Do not use if patient needs restricted sodium intake	
Ethionamide	10-15 mg/kg, not to exceed 1.0 gram	Gastrointestinal: anorexia, nausea, vomiting		Divided dose may help control gastrointestinal side effects	Protein Synthesis (Bacteriocidal)
		Hepatotoxicity	SGOT, SGPT	Discontiune if SGOT is more than twice normal or jaundice develops	
		Postural hypotension, depression, asthenia, drowsiness			
		Skin rash, purpura, gynecomastia, impotence			

(cont'd.)

DRUG	DOSE	SIDE EFFECTS	MONITORING	REMARKS	SITE OF ACTION
Pyrazinamide	40-50 mg/kg not to exceed 3.0 grams per day in 3 divided doses	Hyperuricemia: acute gout	Uric acid		Unknown (Bacteriostatic)
		Hepatotoxicity	SGOT, SGPT	More common with high dosage	
		Gastrointestinal: anorexia, nausea			
		Diabetes mellitus more difficult to manage			
Cycloserine	15 mg/kg not to exceed 1.0 gram in 3-4 divided doses	Central Nervous System: somnolence, headache, tremor, dysarthria, vertigo, agitated depression, psychosis, seizures	Clinical follow-up of neurologic and psychologic status	More common with higher dosage and in presence of ethanol. Serum levels may help. Anticonvulsants have been used to control seizures	Cell Wall Synthesis (Bacteriostatic)

		Hypersensitivity: rash			
Strepto-mycin	15 mg/kg not to exceed 1.0 gram in single daily dose for 2-3 months, then 3 times/week	8th cranial nerve damage	Audiogram, tinnitus, hearing loss. Vestibular function: vertigo	Use with caution in presence of renal insufficiency and in older patients	Protein Synthesis (Bacteriocidal)
		Nephrotoxicity	BUN, creatinine	Rare	
		Neuromuscular junction blockade		Seen in patients also receiving muscle relaxants or with myasthenia gravis	
		Hypersensitivity reactions: rash, dermatitis, anaphylaxis		Rare	
		Skin rash			

(cont'd.)

DRUG	DOSE	SIDE EFFECTS	MONITORING	REMARKS	SITE OF ACTION
Kanamycin	15 mg/kg not to exceed 1.0 gram in single dose, 5 times/ week	8th cranial nerve damage	Audiogram, tinnitus, hearing loss. Vestibular function: vertigo	Same as with streptomycin	Protein Synthesis (Bacteriocidal)
		Nephrotoxicity	BUN, creatinine		
		Hypersensitivity reactions: rash, pruritus			
		Neuromuscular junction blockade			
Viomycin	15 mg/kg not to exceed 1.0 gram in single daily dose	8th cranial nerve damage	Audiogram, tinnitus, hearing loss. Vestibular function: vertigo	Same as for streptomycin	Protein Synthesis (Bacteriocidal)
		Nephrotoxicity	BUN, creatinine		

		Hypersensitivity: rash, urticaria			
		Electrolyte imbalance		Watch for muscle weakness, tetany due to urinary loss of calcium, potassium & chloride & retention of bicarbonate	
Capreomycin	15 mg/kg not to exceed 1.0 g in single daily dose	8th cranial nerve damage	Audiogram, tinnitus, hearing loss. Vestibular function: vertigo	Same as for streptomycin	Protein Synthesis (Bacteriocidal)
		Nephrotoxicity	BUN, creatinine, urinalysis		
		Hypokalemia	Serum potassium		
		Hypersensitivity reactions: rash, urticaria, eosinophilia			
		Neuromuscular junction blockade			

APPENDIX 3

SIGNIFICANT DRUG RESISTANCE LEVELS IN DIRECT DRUG SUSCEPTIBILITY STUDIES ON 7H11 MEDIA*	
Isoniazid	0. 2-1. 0**
Streptomycin	2. 0
Ethambutol	5. 0-10. 0**
Rifampin	1. 0-5. 0-10. 0**
Para-aminosalicylic acid	5. 0
Ethionamide	5. 0-10. 0**
Cycloserine	30. 0
Kanamycin	5. 0
Viomycin	5. 0
Capreomycin	10. 0

**Growth at lower concentration indicates probable resistance and at the higher level definite resistance.

*Taken from: Treatment of Pulmonary Tuberculosis. Byrd RB, Kaplan PD, Gracey DR. <u>Chest</u> 66:560-567, 1974.

APPENDIX 4

MYCOBACTERIAL CHARACTERISTICS

GROUP	PIGMENT	CATALASE	NIACIN
M. Tuberculosis (susceptible)	None	+	+
M. Tuberculosis (INH Resistant)	None	-	+
I. Photochromogens	Yellow	+	-
II. Scotochromogens	Yellow	+	-
III. Nonchromogens	None	-	-
IV. Rapid Growers	Variable	-	-

INDEX

INDEX

Acid-fast bacilli, 5
Adrenal insufficiency, 38
Antituberculous drugs
action of, 25
dose, 96
interactions, 27
side effects, 25
therapy, 29
use of, 30
Appendices, 93
Atypical mycobacteria
classification, 94, 107
See Mycobacterioses, 69

BCG vaccination, 21
Bacteriology, 2
Biopsy
pleural, 9, 10
tissue, 9

CNS tuberculosis, 36
Chemotherapy, 1
doses, 96
drug resistant cases, 61
practice of, 29
retreatment, 64
supervised, 63
supervised intermittent therapy, 39, 55
Children
treatment of tuberculosis in, 31
Concentric Circle
approach to contact evaluation, 19
Classification, 1, 93, 94
Contact Evaluation, 18
case, 43
"concentric circle", 19
method, 18
Corticosteroids
adjunct to treatment, 38
INH preventive therapy and, 17

Diet, 1
Droplet nuclei, 5
M. tuberculosis, 5
Drug action, 25

Extrapulmonary tuberculosis, 35
CNS, 36
genitourinary, 36
miliary, 37
skeletal, 36, 50
treatment, 35

Fever, 34

Gastric washing
cultures, 7
stains (AFB), 8, 10
Genitourinary tuberculosis, 36
Granulomas
caseating, 5

Heliotherapy, 1
Hemoptysis, 34
treatment, 35
Hepatitis
INH induced, 14, 15, 26

Immune mechanisms, 5
Infection
acquired, 5
progressive primary, 6
reactivation, 6
Intermittent drug therapy, 1, 2, 39, 55
Isoniazid, 6
contraindications, 20
induced hepatitis, 14, 21

preventive therapy, 14, 19

Medical surveillance
discharge from, 31
Miliary tuberculosis, 37
Mucociliary clearance, 5
Mycobacteria
culturing, 2, 5, 7, 8
sensitivity, drug, 2
staining, 2, 8
Mycobacterioses, 69
classification, 69, 94
M. tuberculosis
drug resistance, 24
infection, 5, 10
nature of, 24
number of organisms, 24
skin test, 6, 13
staining, 8, 9, 10
treatment, 24

Nontuberculous septicemia, 34

Patient
characteristics, 28
Phagocytosis, 6
Pleural fluid
cultures, 8
stains, 8
Pneumothorax, 1
Preventive therapy, 6
adverse effects, 14
alcoholism and, 20
contraindications, 20
current guidelines, 14
evaluation of candidates, 19
follow-up of, 20
indications for, 14
isoniazid, 6, 19
monitoring, 20
other medications and, 20
pregnancy and, 20
Progressive primary infection, 6

Ranke complex
with Ghon lesion, 14
Reactivation, 1, 2, 3, 6
Respiratory bronchiole, 5
Respiratory failure, 33
Reistant tuberculosis, 60
primary type, 60
secondary (acquired), 60
Retreatment, 2, 64
Roentgenographic appearance, 2

Sarcoid
granulomas, 12
Short-term therapy, 1, 2
Skeletal tuberculosis, 36
Skin test
anergy, 6, 7
"booster effect", 7, 17
classification of results, 13
conversion, 16
effect of blood transfusion, 17
"false-negative", 6, 7
"false-positive", 7, 17
interpretation, 13
Mantoux, 13
Monovac, 13
technique, 13
Tine, 13
tuberculin, 6, 13
Sputum
cultures, 7
induction, 7
positivity, 18
Surgery, 1, 87
Surgical treatment, 87

Tissue biopsy, 5
Treatment
drug, 1, 2, 24
duration, 25
failure, 2, 3

of drug resistant TB, 60
retreatment, 64
Tuberculosis
categorization of, 29, 93
classification, 93
complications of, 33
diagnosis of, 2, 5
dissemination, 35
drug resistant, 60
endobronchial, 38
extrapulmonary, 35
fever in, 34
pulmonary, 3, 40, 45
retreatment, 64
surgical treatment, 87
treatment, 29, 39, 40, 45, 55
treatment of children, 31

Tween 80 stabilized PPD, 6

Urine
cultures, 8